Encounters
with
Qi

W·W·NORTON & COMPANY
New York   London

Encounters with Qi

Exploring Chinese Medicine

DAVID EISENBERG, M.D.
with
THOMAS LEE WRIGHT

First published as a Norton paperback 1995

The text of this book is composed in Bodoni Book.
Composition and manufacturing by The Haddon Craftsmen, Inc.
Book design by Jacques Chazaud.

Library of Congress Cataloging in Publication Data
Eisenberg, David, M.D.
    Encounters with qi.
    Includes index.
    1. Medicine, Chinese. 2. Vital force. I. Wright,
Thomas. II. Title. [DNLM: 1. Medicine, Oriental
Traditional—China. WB 50 JC6 E3e]
R602.E4 1985   610   85–4921

ISBN 0-393-31213-5

W. W. Norton & Company, Inc.
500 Fifth Avenue, New York, N.Y. 10110
W. W. Norton & Company Ltd.
10 Coptic Street, London WC1A 1PU

1 2 3 4 5 6 7 8 9 0

To my mother,
Dorothy Eisenberg

Contents

Foreword

David Eisenberg and I met as student and teacher in my course in behavioral medicine at the Harvard Medical School. Dr. Eisenberg was at that time already keenly interested in China and its traditional medical practices. As you will see in the pages that follow, he soon put his interest to the practical test of travel and study in China. Because of my own research into a wide range of mind-body interactions, and the alternative medical systems based on them, I was eager to hear about Dr. Eisenberg's observations. I was especially curious about Qi Gong and the mind-body interactions which underlie so much of Chinese medicine. Eventually he and I visited China together to view Qi Gong activities and to study its practitioners. That research continues today, and Dr. Eisenberg is now my colleague in the Division of Behavioral Medicine at the Harvard Medical School.

Chinese traditional medicine, the Ayurvedic medicine of India, Tibetan medicine, and other Eastern medical systems evolved, for the most part, independently of Western scientific medicine. Until the twentieth century the Eastern and Western medical systems were each considered particularly efficacious by their own practitioners. Today, Western medicine is generally believed to be the standard of excellence against which all other practices should be judged.

The exalted position of Western scientific medicine is justified because it effects so many cures not possible by the others. Yet it was not always in such a leadership role. Prior to the twentieth century, Western medicine was, by today's standards, of questionable worth. L. J. Henderson, one of Harvard's notable biochemists, is said to have stated, "Sometime between 1910 and 1912 in this country, a random patient, with a random disease, consulting a doctor chosen at random, had, for the first time in the history of mankind, a better than fifty-fifty chance of profiting from the encounter."

The success of treatments before the twentieth century was related to nonspecific or placebo effects. A placebo, as Dr. A. K. Shapiro has written, is any treatment or aspect of treatment that does not have a specific action on a patient's disorder or symptoms. But placebos are not limited to sugar pills and other inactive substances. Any nonspecific aspect of treatment is a placebo and includes the mind-sets of both patients and doctors. Three major elements are necessary to bring forth the effects of placebos: the beliefs and expectations of the patient, the beliefs and expectations of the doctor, and the doctor-patient relationship. All these factors are at work in Chinese and other non-Western medical practices.

In the course of the twentieth century, Western medicine defined specific therapies. Antibiotics were discovered. Prior to the use of antibiotics which rendered the causative agent of tuberculosis innocuous, this disease was rampant. In fact, before the 1950s most hospital beds in the United States were devoted to the care of patients suffering from tuberculosis. After the discovery and widespread use of penicillin, pneumonia was no longer the dreaded disease it had once been. Syphilis, gonorrhea, and other severe infections also became curable. Insulin was isolated; it could correct diabetes and its severe, life-threatening manifestations. Vitamins became understood, and their use could cure pellagra, rickets, beriberi, and scurvy. Surgery was able to effectively restore traumatized bodies. Sight could be returned to patients with cataracts. Infants born with heart defects could have surgical correction in early childhood and live normal lives. The list goes on and is extensive and impressive. These treatments were successful whether or not they were believed in, even in the presence of an unsympathetic physician.

The importance and worth of the nonspecific treatments or placebo effects were minimized alongside these new powerful, indeed, wonderous, specific treatments. These therapies had awesome success and remarkable consistency when compared with those of the placebo effect. The placebo effect became a ridiculed aspect of treatment. It could not compete successfully. Many of its worthwhile aspects were abandoned, and Western medicine came to depend, almost exclusively, on specific therapies. The therapies of non-Western medicine, which are often nonspecific, were deemed unworthy of attention.

However, at present only about 25 percent of the illnesses that bring a Western patient to a Western physician are successfully treated by specific agents and procedures. The other 75 percent either get better by themselves or are related to nonspecific, mind-body interactions. Our Western medical approach is thus rather limited in its efficacy. We cannot afford to ignore other medical practices. We should investigate them and determine what is specific and nonspecific. We should then incorporate the useful features into our Western practice and share our own knowledge with the practitioners of alternative systems.

As the twentieth century draws to a close, China faces a historic choice. How will it preserve the riches of its traditional medicine while embracing the specific technologies and interventions of Western medicine? For our own part, we in the West are now looking more carefully, and less condescendingly, at alternative practices of medicine and mind-body interactions. We are using scientific technologies to investigate nonspecific therapies and placebo effects. *Encounters with Qi,* with its entertaining and instructive descriptions of traditional Chinese medicine, is a pioneering contribution to mutual understanding between East and West. Only David Eisenberg could have written this fine account.

Herbert Benson, M.D.
Boston, June 1985

Acknowledgments

A Yuan dynasty proverb says, "A teacher for a day is to be respected like a father for a lifetime." I have had the good fortune of meeting many excellent teachers at the Harvard Medical School, and am particularly indebted to Drs. H. Richard Nesson, Robert Lawrence, Daniel Federman, Dieter Koch-Weser, Leon Eisenberg, Arthur Kleinman, and Herbert Benson. This book, in many ways, is a tribute to their curiosity, scholarship, encouragement, and support.

I thank the U.S. National Academy of Sciences Committee on Scholarly Communications with the People's Republic of China for the opportunity to live, work, and study in Beijing. I am also grateful to the Harvard Medical School International Medical Programs Office, the Paul Dudley White Memorial Foundation, and the Harvard Medical School Division of Behavioral Medicine for financial support of my research.

I am indebted to the following Chinese medical authorities for reviewing the manuscript prior to its publication: Dr. Wu Jie-ping, president, Chinese Academy of Medical Sciences; Dr. Xie Zhu-fan, director of traditional medicine, Beijing Medical College; Dr. Lu Zhi-jun, president, All-China Society of Acupuncture and Moxibustion; Dr. Shi Yu-shu, professor, Tian Jin Medical College; Dr. Lin Ya-gu, director, Shanghai Qi Gong Research Institute; Dr. Shen Jia-qi, superintendent, Shanghai Qi Gong Research Institute; Dr. Wang Yu-ren, president, Shanghai Institute of Traditional Chinese Medicine.

My thanks to the UCLA Department of Internal Medicine for permitting me to continue my China research during my residency training. My special thanks to Dr. K. Kit Hui, internist, clinical pharmacologist, and scholar of Chinese medicine, for teaching me so much about the integration of Chinese and Western medical practice. To Drs. Kenneth Shine, Dennis Cope, Roy Young, Neil Parker, Marvin Derezin, David Rimer, Joseph Perloff, Herbert Weiner, and Joel Yager, I express my sincerest thanks for their valuable support.

My thanks to Eric Ashworth of Candida Donadio and Associates, for believing in the merits of an unfinished manuscript by an unpublished author, and for finding a home for this book. Hilary Hinzmann at W. W. Norton & Co., Inc. helped refine the ideas in this book and skillfully edited the manuscript.

Other people who helped in the early development of this book include Patty Johnston, Robert Gordon, Andrew Gellis, Matthew Rushton, James Feinerman, Carola Eisenberg, Victoria Trembley, Howard Sawyer, Ivy Lin, Bonnie Glasberg, David Maron, Elliott Fisher, Nan Cochran, Carla Millhauser, and Sandra Wright.

I thank my Chinese hosts, teachers, and friends for their generosity and kindness. Wang Jin-huai, a calligrapher and scholar of Chinese medicine, helped me appreciate the importance of Qi. Together with Dr. Ren Ying-qiu and Dr. Lu Bing-kuai, he introduced me to many of the Qi-related phenomena described in this book. To my friends Cai Hong, Sun Li-zhe, Huang Shan, Li Shi-zhuo, Rong Bing-lan, Yang Shu-lian, Fang Chi, and Fei Li-min, I express my deepest thanks for their assistance.

Thomas Wright, my college classmate and close friend, encouraged me to write this book and spent the next five years patiently guiding me through every stage of its development. His literary insight has helped shape this book from start to finish.

I am especially grateful to my friend and teacher Dr. Ma Hai De (George Hatem), the American-born, Western-trained senior adviser to the Chinese Ministry of Health. Since 1935 George Hatem has been a limitless source of inspiration for the Chinese people and for all friends of China.

Finally, I wish to acknowledge the unconditional support of my loving family.

Encounters
with
Qi

The Woman
on the Bus

After visiting friends at Beijing University, I waited for the last bus of the night. As the empty No. 107 pulled up, three Chinese teenagers jumped ahead of the line, wrestled their way to the side door, and leaped inside. I took a window seat and turned to watch the other passengers climb aboard.

A young woman in khaki trousers and white shirt, her hair in pigtails, struggled to climb the stairs at the rear door. She took a step at a time, leaning on the forearm of a handsome factory worker who, after helping her to a seat a few rows behind me, stood vigil with arms folded in his blue, neatly pressed Mao jacket.

The doors closed, and we were off into the quiet night. The electric bus carried us onto a dusty roadway.

We had traveled only a short distance when the woman let out a moan. She put her hands to her face and began to sob quietly.

As the factory worker moved closer, the woman grasped his arm, buried her face in his sleeve, and cried.

This was the first time I had seen a Chinese cry in public. Some people on the bus, wishing to spare the woman embarrassment, moved away from her, changed seats, or looked in another direction. Two young men weren't so considerate. They wore poorly fitted Western bell-bottoms, long hair (by Chinese standards), and dark sunglasses imported from Hong Kong. They stared menacingly at the woman through blue-tinted lenses, which still sported the manufacturer's label. The factory worker arched his back, looking directly into those absurd sunglasses and making clear that these "bad eggs" had best conform to propriety. In reply, one of the boys hawked and spit on the bus floor just inches from my shoe, produced a pack of cigarettes and offered a butt to the other one. Then they adjusted their glasses, put their hands in their jacket pockets, and sauntered to the far end of the bus.

By now the woman was crying uncontrollably, her moans broken by gasping, brief silences and the whirring of the electric bus engine.

I wondered whether I should offer assistance—Should a foreigner intrude in this sort of situation?—but I felt that something had to be done. Adjusting the school pin on my lapel— in Chinese, "Beijing Institute of Traditional Chinese Medicine" —I got up from my seat to face the factory worker. Should I introduce myself as I would in the United States or should I approach the patient in the style of a typical Chinese doctor by asking, "You have what illness?" I opted for diplomacy.

"Hello, I'm an American doctor working at the Institute of Traditional Chinese Medicine. You have what illness?"

"Legs," the unnerved woman replied. She explained in gasps that she felt excruciating pain in the bones of her legs. It had begun just before she climbed aboard the bus. She felt weak, and the weakness was becoming total paralysis. She could not move her legs and had no sensation from the thighs downward. She sucked in a breath of air and winced with pain. The factory worker hugged her tightly to muffle the crying in his coat.

"This is my younger sister."

"Has she suffered these attacks before?"

"Only this past year. Never this severe."

He was frightened.

"The pains are getting worse little by little," the young woman pleaded. "What can be done?"

I felt ill equipped to diagnose this woman's trouble. I was, after all, a fourth-year medical student, not a board-certified neurologist. I asked whether she could move her legs or feet. She could not. I pinched her leg, but she felt nothing. I removed my school pin and poked her repeatedly with the sharp end of the needle. She felt no sensation. Her pupils, her pulse, and her respiration were all normal.

This woman needed to be seen in an emergency room right away. She resisted, but her brother agreed with me and asked for directions to the nearest hospital. I offered to escort them to the Dong Zhi Men Hospital at my institute, only one stop away. The brother carried her the first few blocks, but the emergency room was half a mile from the bus stop, and he soon agreed to let me carry her so he could catch his breath.

Then an army jeep drove up the road. I waved it down as the brother tugged at my sleeve, imploring me to leave the army out of this business.

"It's not their responsibility," he said.

I paid no attention, though it was clear the brother feared he would be criticized for involving the army in a personal problem. Five People's Liberation Army soldiers were in the jeep. Their commander, sitting in the passenger seat, asked me what the trouble was.

"This woman is ill. We need to get her to the Dong Zhi Men emergency room immediately."

The commander ordered the soldiers to lend a hand. The woman was dazed, no longer responding to questions, as we lifted her gently onto the backseat. We stood on the floorboards while the jeep sped off toward the main gate of the hospital.

An old sign pointed to the emergency-room entrance, but because bricks and lumber blocked the road, we reversed direction to look for another route. About two hundred yards from the emergency entrance, we parked in a trench. There were no lights. I jumped off the jeep into ankle-deep mud and ran to the building with the woman's brother.

In the dark hallway, Chinese peasants waited quietly on wooden benches. Nurses bandaged an unconscious elderly woman with gauze cloths from an old wooden cart.

The emergency-room orderlies recognized my badge and referred me to a nearby nursing station. I let the brother do the talking as we requested a stretcher. The head nurse looked down her nose at us.

"Who is it for?"

The brother said his sister was outside in the jeep.

"Hospital policy says a patient can use a stretcher only after signing in at the desk."

The brother pointed out that his sister would be unable to sign in unless we carried her in on the stretcher.

The nurse smiled, as if to say, "I'm just following the rules." Catch-22.

Perhaps out of politeness to a foreigner, the head nurse let me vouch for the stretcher until the patient could sign herself in.

Back at the jeep the young woman was still in apparent pain;

though her vital signs were normal, she was moaning incessantly. After the soldiers placed her on the stretcher and drove off, we toted her over rubble to the emergency room, where the physician-on-call was now waiting.

He wore a long white lab coat over his gray Mao jacket, a tieless white shirt closed to the top button, and thick horn-rimmed glasses. In the upper lab coat pocket, he kept a set of acupuncture needles. Additional needles were laid out on a nearby tray. There were no stethoscopes or ophthalmoscopes—just needles. I wondered whether the doctor's skills in traditional Chinese medicine would enable him to handle this emergency.

The doctor assessed the situation by observing the woman's interaction with her brother. He turned to the brother, without preliminary questions, and asked, "Is she hysterical?"

I began to regret that we hadn't taken this young woman to a Western-style hospital close by.

The woman declared that she was not hysterical. The doctor acted as if he didn't care what she had to say. To my surprise, he took out a reflex hammer and proceeded to test her reflexes: response normal.

The doctor told the woman she needed acupuncture, and she moaned in reply. He carefully selected four extremely fine three-inch needles. He inserted a needle between and parallel to the first and second toe of each foot, to a depth of half an inch. He inserted two additional needles into points located in the middle of each sole, twisting these needles in by hand, perpendicular to the skin, to a depth of nearly an inch. These rarely used points are classic for the acupuncture treatment of hysteria, having been used for thousands of years, and are normally quite painful. In this case, however, the woman felt nothing at all.

The Chinese doctor stood at her feet and twisted the needles into her soles. Holding the ends of the needles between thumb and forefinger, he rolled them back and forth three or four times per second, inserting and withdrawing them at various angles to stimulate the acupuncture points.

As each needle was inserted, the doctor asked, *"De Qi le mei you?"*

I had never heard this expression before. The word *Qi* (气, pronounced "chēē") means "vital energy." Each time the doctor jabbed the woman with a needle, he was asking, "Do you feel the vital energy?" If she said yes, he left the needle where it was and twisted it back and forth. If she answered no, he withdrew it and tried again at a slightly different angle. This was repeated with each needle until the young woman said, *"De le"* ("I've got it").

Within thirty seconds, the young woman reported slight sensations in her feet. After a minute or so, she could wiggle her toes. When three minutes had passed, she complained that the needles in her soles were exquisitely painful and asked that they be removed. The doctor then twisted and jabbed the needles between her first and second toes. In less than seven minutes, she regained full motor and sensory function. The needles were removed, and she was allowed off the stretcher to walk around.

She shuffled around like a person whose legs have gone to sleep. As she walked, she complained. This bizarre paralysis had afflicted her no fewer than six times in the past year. Headaches, backaches, and weakness had laid her low. Her fiancé had left her. Her superiors at the crafts factory did not like her work, and she could not find another job.

The Chinese doctor interrupted her, "You should not become so anxious. You ought to relax more. And it is absolutely essential for your medical condition that you lead a happy life." With this admonition, he handed her a prescription for eight herbs.

26

When the woman left the room, I asked the Chinese doctor what he had prescribed.

"A tranquilizer," he said, turning to face me. "And tell me, do you have patients in your country who need tranquilizers?"

Preface

This book is based on my trips to China in the period from 1977 through 1985. I made most of the observations while working inside urban Chinese hospitals in 1979 and 1980, though the path that led me to the East began earlier.

When the *New York Times* columnist James Reston underwent an appendectomy while accompanying the Nixon entourage to Beijing in 1971, he wrote about a medical discovery called "acupuncture anesthesia." Reston's account of this innovation changed the course of my medical education and prompted me to find out everything I could about China and its medicine.

I was in my freshman year at Harvard when I began to study the Chinese language. By the time I graduated, I had read the handful of books describing the fundamentals of traditional Chinese medicine. Courses with John King Fairbank and other scholars had opened up to me China's rich past and its turbulent present. I was fascinated by what China might teach the West. Descriptions of the Chinese health care system* suggested that it was among the most progressive in the world.

In 1976 I hoped to win a fellowship to study medicine in the People's Republic, but in the absence of formal U.S.-Chinese diplomatic relations, no foundations would assist me. In 1977, after my first year at Harvard Medical School, I traveled to Taipei, Taiwan, improving my language skills and observing acupuncturists, herbalists, massage therapists, and faith healers.

In 1978 I accompanied a Harvard Medical School delegation on a tour of hospitals in Beijing and Shanghai. Six months later the United States established diplomatic relations with the People's Republic of China, and within weeks the U.S. National Academy of Sciences advertised for graduate students fluent in Chinese to serve as exchange scholars. I was selected as the first American medical exchange student to the People's Republic of China and took a leave of absence from medical school to study medicine in Beijing for a full year—August 1979 through August 1980.

When I returned to the United States, my views were further shaped by residency training in internal medicine at the UCLA Medical Center. As an internist and clinical research fellow at the Harvard Medical School, I have continued my study of the practices of Chinese physicians.

In 1983 I returned to the People's Republic with a medical delegation whose primary objective was to study the most fundamental and baffling element of Chinese medicine—Qi, the concept of "vital energy."

---

* See, for example, Joshua S. Horn, *Away with All Pests: An English Surgeon in People's China, 1954–1969* (New York: Monthly Review Press, 1971), and Victor W. Sidel and Ruth Sidel, *Serve the People: Observations on Medicine in the People's Republic of China* (Boston: Beacon Press, 1973).

This book describes what I learned and poses some large questions:

- What can we in the West learn from the medical practices of the Chinese people that might improve our understanding of health, illness, and the healing process?
- Which Chinese medical techniques should we investigate?
- Can Chinese medicine be integrated into Western medical practices?
- Can Chinese medicine prove its assertion that life-style and attitude can significantly alter the natural course of human illness?

My encounters with Qi satisfied my curiosity—and frustrated it, in unexpected ways. I offer them here as a first step toward a more complete understanding of traditional Chinese medicine.

First Encounter:
Dr. Fang
and the Yellow
Emperor

During my first weeks in Beijing I caused quite a stir. My blue eyes, curly blond hair, and beard marked me as a foreign curiosity. Adults reacted as if confronted by an alien from another planet. Infants were mesmerized and horrified. On a street corner, a group of schoolchildren gently took hold of my arms and walked me across the street. Having noticed my blue-gray eyes, they assumed I was totally blind and wanted to escort me through the traffic. In the marketplace, a distinguished gentleman introduced himself in broken English as an ophthalmologist. He then asked politely whether he could study my eyes. He had never examined blue eyes before. Because of my beard, people assumed I was older than my twenty-four years. Young women thought my hair was dyed and permed. Most days I wore a gray Mao jacket, worker's pants, and yellow Brooks running shoes. Everyone loved the shoes.

At first I lived at the Beijing Foreign Language Institute preparing for traditional medical school, where every class was taught in the Mandarin language. Mornings I awoke to nearly total quiet. No car horns. No dogs barking—they had been done away with in public-health campaigns years ago. Outside my window, black smoke billowed from the coal stoves of the dining halls. Students were outside by 5:30 A.M., exercising, jogging, practicing martial arts, or playing basketball. Some paced back and forth, reciting language lessons. A monotonous drone of mispronounced tongues, from English to Arabic, blended with the sound of bouncing basketballs.

My morning meals consisted of tea and a fried dough stick or a bowl of rice porridge. For the first time, my personal belongings were few, my room uncluttered, my desk empty except for a Cross pen and airmail stationery from home. I had a couple of books, a change of clothes or two, no telephone, and lots of time to myself.

A Chinese maxim says that physicians ought to be exemplary physical specimens. My spare time gave me the opportunity to live up to this sensible ideal by running regularly and studying Tai Ji Quan (sometimes called Tai Chi).

I ran each day at sunset. At first it was work, but it soon became an addiction. By steadily increasing my mileage from three to five to ten miles a day, I covered a lot of countryside. I ran from my small room at the institute, through a market and commune, to a factory near Beijing University, through rice fields and cabbage fields on rural back roads, often stopping at beautiful Kun-Ming Lake below the Summer Palace grounds. I introduced myself to people along the way. Friends called me Dr. Ai (short for *Ai Sen Bo*). Local peasants came out as I ran by, waiting at sunset like clockwork. The brickmakers called out, *"Quai yi diar Lao Ai"* ("A little faster, Old Ai"). Bakers at the bread factory invited me to stop for tea and bread. Children from the orchard sat in tree houses and screamed, *"Ai dai fu lai le, Ai dai fu lai le!"* ("Doctor Ai has come again, Doctor Ai has come again!"). On sunny afternoons, an eighty-nine-year-old farmer named Zhang sat on his wood-carved stool next to the ice-stick stand at the foot of the Summer Palace. Zhang always waved as I went by, then made a fist and stuck his thumb in the air with a smile. Even the tough-looking security guards at the railroad crossings waited for me to appear. For my benefit, they whistled "Yankee Doodle Dandy," the theme song of the newly broadcast Voice of America radio show.

My spartan surroundings and rigorous exercise schedule began to cause changes in my body. I lost ten pounds, and my resting pulse dropped from seventy to fifty. I felt as if my body and my mind were functioning on a new level. What had happened? Was my well-being attributable to the training effects of exercise? What about the influence of my altered diet, which consisted mainly of rice and vegetables and included little meat or fat? Perhaps it was due to stress reduction in my move from Harvard Medical School to the outskirts of Beijing. Maybe the study of Asian philosophies had altered my belief system sufficiently to change my health.

Whatever the cause, I felt immeasurably better than I had when I left the United States certified "healthy." Perhaps back then I had not been "healthy" so much as "not sick."

When it was nearly winter in northern China, the daily Beijing newspapers warned of "big Siberian winds." These remnants of the Ice Age came by way of northern Russia and Mongolia. Air temperatures of ten to twenty degrees Fahrenheit rode in on sixty-mile-per-hour winds.

The day of my transfer from the Beijing Foreign Language Institute to the Institute of Traditional Chinese Medicine, I wore woolen long underwear, three pair of socks, two turtlenecks, a sweater, flannel trousers, a down vest, hat, gloves, boots, and my oversize, ankle-length padded coat.

At the Institute of Traditional Chinese medicine, the living conditions resembled those at the Language Institute. Hot water was available only for an hour or two on certain days. The nearest toilet or sink was a hundred yards from my room. Whenever more than two people plugged in shortwave radios or portable stoves, sparks flew and fuses blew.

The difficult conditions did not diminish the positive aspects of my transfer. Instead of living in a dormitory complex fifteen miles outside the city, I had moved into a tranquil two-hundred-year-old traditional Chinese courtyard located one mile from the center of the city. The Beijing Institute of Traditional Chinese Medicine is one of five key centers of higher traditional medical education in China—an ideal place for a foreign student to receive a medical education unavailable in the West.

Being the first American medical exchange student gave me certain advantages. I was assigned the finest teachers, a custom-tailored curriculum, and one-on-one tutorials exclusively.

My professors spoke no English. Their medicine was based on three thousand years of observation and philosophy, not on the scientific method of my Harvard medical instructors. My Western training relied heavily on causal relations, structure, and quantitative changes. The Chinese, by contrast, recognized patterns defined by a circular system of logic. We were worlds apart, but we would come together for a short time to share what we knew about health and illness.

The nonclinical tutorials took place in a small room in a distant courtyard of the institute. The room had two hard chairs, a worn desk, and a broken blackboard. The window was boarded up. There was no heat or fireplace. For four hours every morning

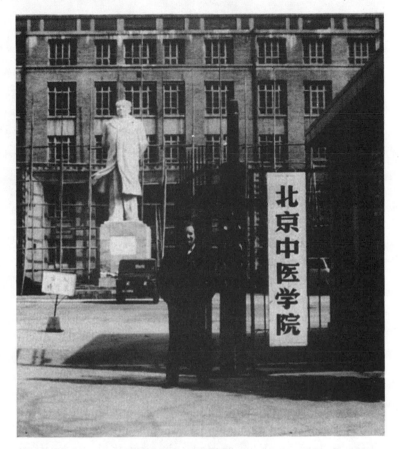

The author, at the Beijing Institute of Traditional Chinese Medicine.

and three hours in the afternoon, I sat face to face with my teachers in the cold. While they lectured, I took notes.

In these talks the names of Hippocrates, Galen, or Pasteur never came up. Instead, I learned about the forefathers of traditional Chinese medicine. For instance, there was the Yellow Emperor, believed to have lived from ca. 2700 to ca. 2600 B.C., whose name is synonymous with the most famous treatise of Chinese medicine—the *Neijing* (Classic of Internal Medicine).* Nearly three thousand years later, in the third century A.D., Wang Shu-he wrote a treatise on pulse diagnosis. And in the sixteenth century Li Shi-jen catalogued more than 12,000 recipes for preparing herbal medications.

My class on Chinese medical theory was taught by Doctor Fang, a practitioner of traditional medicine for twenty years. Fang was professor of traditional Chinese medical theory. His expertise was "Yin and Yang Theory," "The Five Elements," "The Organ Systems," and "The Origins of Qi."

A stocky man in his forties, Fang had large shoulders, a round face, a crewcut, 1950s-style thick black eyeglasses, and six gold-capped front teeth. Fang grew up in a small city in Shanxi Province a few hundred miles from Beijing. The men in his family had been doctors of traditional medicine for more than six generations. Although proud of this fact, he was quick to point out that a colleague in the Department of Herbal Medicine knew the names of physicians in his family for *nineteen* generations.

Each morning around seven-thirty Fang rode up to my courtyard on his Shanghai-built industrial-strength bicycle. Its tires and shocks enabled it to haul pigs, concrete blocks, or two adults sitting on the rear. Fang carried only a small plastic briefcase that held his books and a teacup with a lid. As we discussed theories and philosophies, he chain-smoked hand-rolled ciga-

---

* The legendary Yellow Emperor is actually a composite of numerous ancient physicians. Written by many scholars in the third or second century B.C., the *Neijing* summarized the theoretical and practical knowledge of prior centuries. Translations here are by the author, based on Ilza Veith's translation, *The Yellow Emperor's Classic of Internal Medicine* (Berkeley: University of California Press, 1966).

rettes and sipped jasmine tea. We broke for a walk around the courtyard every two hours.

Fang began our first meeting with a discussion of the ancient Daoist origins of Yin and Yang. According to traditional medicine, the principle of Yin and Yang is the basis of the entire universe: "It is the principle of everything in Creation. It is the source of life and death."

Fang elaborated, "Yin and Yang represent opposing yet complementary aspects of the universe. For example, that which is cold is Yin, that which is hot is Yang. Night is Yin, day is Yang, and so on. Every object, every action, every aspect of time and space, can be thought of in terms of a preponderance of either Yin or Yang. And within Yang there is something of Yin. For example, the roof of a house is Yang (up) relative to the ground, but Yin (down) relative to the stars. Nothing exists that is neither Yin nor Yang, and all natural events are influenced by the constantly changing relationships of these two formless aspects of all things."

"Can the human biological processes also be thought of in terms of Yin and Yang?" I asked.

"The solid organs are said to be Yin, and the hollow organs are Yang. Female is Yin, male is Yang. Chronic diseases are Yin, while acute diseases are Yang."

When viewed in these terms, the body, like the universe, is a complex system of Yin and Yang. Yin and Yang ebb and flow, changing through constant motion. One can give rise to or be diminished by the other. According to Chinese medicine, a balance of Yin and Yang results in health; an imbalance leads to disease.

"What about a piece of chalk?" I asked. "Is it Yin or Yang?"

"It has characteristics of both Yin and Yang," Fang said. "Because it is dry, it is Yang. Because it is white, it is Yin. Its

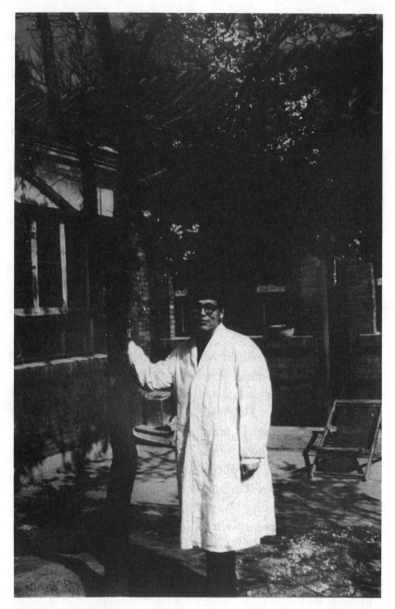

Dr. Fang, a specialist in Chinese medical theory.

surface is Yang because its exterior is Yang, but its interior aspect is Yin. This piece of chalk, like all the universe, is a mixture of Yin and Yang."

"This system is confusing to the Western mind."

"Be patient, in time you will understand."

It was first-year medical school all over again. Chinese medical instruction, like Harvard instruction, required the memorization of a large body of information that made little sense at first but that would, I hoped, someday be applicable to my skills as a physician.

After the theory of Yin and Yang, it was time to study the "five elements." According to traditional medicine, everything in the universe, including man, consists of five basic elements: wood, fire, earth, metal, and water. These five elements are subdivisions of Yin and Yang. Everything classified as Yin or Yang also corresponds to one of the five elements. For example, each Yin organ of the body corresponds to one element. In addition, each of the five elements has a corresponding flavor, sound, season, color, direction, weather condition, and the like. Ultimately, every aspect of the universe, including sickness and health, can be analyzed in terms of the five elements.

"Is there any relation," I asked, "between these five elements and their corresponding organs, colors, and smells?"

"Of course," Fang replied. "There is a generating sequence and a subjugating sequence."

"What does that mean?"

"It's quite easy when you think about it. For example, wood destroys earth, earth destroys water, water destroys fire, fire destroys metal, and metal (an axe, for instance) destroys wood. As in all aspects of nature, there are relationships and balances that become clearer when you contemplate them."

"But this is less clear all the time."

"Wood generates fire. Because wood corresponds to the liver and because fire corresponds to the heart, the liver has a generating influence over the heart. In traditional medicine, this is an example of what we call the relationship between 'mother and son.' The organs of the body and all bodily functions are interrelated on the basis of the generating and subjugating sequence of the five elements."

"This is very confusing," I said. "Why should wood correspond to liver and metal to lungs? Do you have proof that this is so? I fail to see how this can have anything to do with the diagnosing or treating of sick people."

"Perhaps you are unclear about these relationships because you do not understand man's relationship to the universe."

"Well, that's not exactly required reading for American medical students."

"Chinese medicine appreciates the relationship between man and nature. Man does not exist in a vacuum. Human life and death are but a minuscule part of the universe and can be influenced by every other aspect of the universe. Life and death are not separate from nature. Furthermore, the laws governing life are the same laws that govern the universe, namely, the ever-changing balance of Yin and Yang. The human body is subject to changes in Yin and Yang. This includes weather, geographic location, seasons, temperature, colors, tastes of foods, and emotions. In short, our bodies are influenced by every aspect of nature.

Fang's words in this first lesson reminded me of the Tai Ji Quan lessons I took from Old Chang, my institute's master. Chang's classes began at six. He was as playful and fit at sixty as a child of eight. Unlike most Chinese men, Old Chang was totally bald. "I have a shiny egg for a head," he would say in his self-deprecating style. "Thank goodness I am already married!" He wore baggy blue cotton sweatsuits over white thermal long johns. His belt was a common piece of cord. This short, raggedly clothed man had the muscles of a gymnast, the grace of a dancer, and the balance of a cat. No ordinary cat, though. Old Chang was a human lion with unmatched power and agility. What's more, he was a scholar.

His appreciation for balance and strength came from a life-long study of Daoist, Confucian, and Buddhist philosophies. The ancient philosophers, who were also China's earliest physicians, had defined the art of Tai Ji Quan in terms that transcended physical discipline. Tai Ji Quan, like all the true martial arts, involved a philosophy of life. The physical discipline of Tai Ji Quan demanded body control and exquisite balance. The movements were slow, circular, symmetrical, and graceful. Performed correctly, they looked effortless.

"Our movements," said Old Chang, "must be like the movements of clouds—constantly changing, but never appearing to change."

"Concentrate on your balance, on left and right, up and down, too much and too little." Here in Old Chang's Tai Ji Quan was a philosophy of Yin and Yang, the two opposite but complementary and interdependent forces of the universe. According to this philosophy, physical exercises were to be guided by a balance of Yin and Yang, just as moral and ethical actions were. Because Yin and Yang were applicable to all aspects of the universe, there was no separation of man from his environment, no Cartesian separation of mind from body. Everything was part of a whole, an unending circle defined by Yin and Yang.

Old Chang insisted we practice every day at sunrise so that we could experience the change in seasons day by day. I had seen the seasons change, of course, but had never paid such close attention to the patterns of the sun, the colors of dawn, and the smells of summer, spring, winter, and fall.

"In a balanced life-style," Chang taught us, "the mind, the body, and the external environment are constantly influencing one another. By neglecting one, you neglect all."

Chang urged us not to hide from the external environment, from the cold of winter, but to continue exercising each morning at dawn whatever the weather. In this way, he said, our bodies would gradually become accustomed to the cold and our minds less afraid of it, and we would ultimately become more resistant to illness.

Fang set human anatomy, a subject I had studied for many years, in a new light: "The human body is composed of Qi, 'vital energy,' channels for the flow of Qi, 'blood,' 'bodily fluids,' 'vital essence,' 'five solid Yin organs,' and 'six hollow Yang organs.' "

This was not the human body as Leonardo da Vinci or *Gray's Medical Anatomy* described it. The organs of Chinese medicine do not correspond precisely to those of Western medicine. For instance, the Chinese concept of the "spleen" is not limited to the mass of tissue in the upper-left corner of the abdomen; it also includes the digestive system as a whole. The "five solid organs" and "six hollow organs" of Chinese medicine are composites of form and function that Daoist philosophers conceived three thousand years ago.*

"The 'solid organs' store 'vital essence,' " Fang said, "and the 'hollow organs' transform the 'essence' and discharge waste. The 'heart,' rather than the brain, as the West believes, is the center of emotional activity and thought processes. Sexual activity is controlled by the 'kidneys.' The 'lungs' are responsible for the

---

* Throughout this book quotation marks are used to indicate anatomy as understood in Chinese medicine.

condition of the skin and hair. The 'heart' is intimately related to the tongue, the 'spleen' to the lips, and the 'kidney' to the ears. In addition, and this will no doubt confuse you more, Dr. Ai, anger and frustration can do pathologic damage to the 'liver,' whereas an abundance of joy will damage the 'heart.' "

The relationships Fang asked me to memorize were different from any taught in Western medical schools. I found it difficult to dissociate myself from my background and my Western biomedical bias. For several weeks, using the cerebral equivalent of brute force, I struggled to memorize these seemingly arbitrary relationships. It was exhausting work. My inability to let go of what I knew—to let go temporarily, at least—made it impossible for me to embrace this bizarre approach to the human body.

"Dr. Ai, you are troubled, are you not?" Fang remarked.

"Yes, very troubled," I replied. "What you have been lecturing about makes so little sense to me. You speak of relationships between specific parts of the human body and nature, relationships between the body and mind that have no basis in Western medicine. Is there some way to tie these relationships together, some concept in Chinese medicine that will help me understand them?"

"Do you understand the meaning of *Qi*—'vital energy'?"

"No, I do not."

"By understanding Qi, Dr. Ai, you will begin to understand much of Chinese medicine. Try and put aside your Western beliefs and do not attempt to compare the concept of Qi to anything you are familiar with."

"I can only try," I said. "What is Qi, really?"

"Qi means that which differentiates life from death, animate from inanimate. To live is to have Qi in every part of your body. To die is to be a body without Qi. For health to be maintained, there must be a balance of Qi, neither too much nor too little.

The origins of Qi are three. There is 'original Qi,' that portion of Qi transmitted from your parents to you. It is unique, yours from the moment of conception. But, it is finite, and over time is used up little by little. The second source of Qi is 'nutritional Qi,' meaning Qi extracted from the food you eat. It is constantly being utilized and replenished. The third is 'air Qi,' the Qi extracted from the air you breathe. It, too, is used and replenished. The function of Qi will help you understand the many relationships you now struggle with. All of human pathology can be seen in terms of balances and imbalances. A balanced state corresponds to health. Any excess or deficiency corresponds to illness. When the body is in a state of equilibrium, internally and with respect to the external environment, then it possesses a 'positive vitality,' a form of Qi that protects the body and defends it from 'pathogenic factors.' "

"In Western terms, could you call this 'resistance' to disease?"

"Precisely. The occurrence of disease is due to the struggle between Qi—vital energy—and 'pathogenic factors.' If the vital energy is insufficient to repulse these 'pathogenic factors,' then the body becomes dysfunctional, and unless treated, this imbalance will result in disease. If the body is imbalanced, then there will be a weakening of 'positive vitality,' and even a minor 'pathogenic factor' can result in illness. Conversely, if one's body is in an excellent state of harmony, then there will be a strong 'positive vitality,' and the most virulent of 'pathogenic factors' will not disturb the body."

The discussion reminded me of a fundamental question in the Western theory of infectious diseases. Given that we are constantly exposed to bacteria and viruses, why don't we become ill from infections all the time? Moreover, given that countless bacteria colonize every human body's skin and gastrointestinal tract, how do we manage to coexist in harmony most of the time but on rare occasions become overwhelmed by these same bacteria? Western medicine has no satisfactory explanation. The concept of "positive vitality" was the Chinese attempt to address this curious aspect of health and illness.

"Dr. Fang," I asked, "where is the Qi and how does it defend the body from 'pathogenic factors'?"

"Qi is in all parts of the body," he explained, "and there is no part which is without Qi. The Qi flows through specific channels—meridians, as you call them. They are conduits connecting all parts of the body. These are the meridians used in acupuncture, and the purpose of acupuncture is simply to reestablish the balance and normal flow of Qi where there is imbalance and stagnation. The purpose of acupressure massage is identical. As for herbal remedies, these are prescribed for the specific purpose of removing any excess or deficiency of Qi. The Qi flows through all internal organs, hollow and solid. Any relative excess or deficiency of Qi will result in disease. This is where the relationships you are struggling to memorize will play a crucial role."

"If there is such a thing as 'positive vitality,' a kind of protective Qi, then what exactly is it protecting against?"

"In Chinese medicine, there are 'pathogenic factors.' These are the elements of life that lead to disease. They include the 'six excesses' (wind, cold, heat, dampness, dryness, and fire), the 'seven moods' (joy, anger, anxiety, obsession, sorrow, horror, and fear), as well as intemperance in eating and drinking, incorrect diet, too much or too little sexual activity, and too much or too little work or exercise. 'Pathogenic factors' can damage parts of the human body and lessen vital energy of the body as a whole. Once an imbalance is created, disease will become manifest. A certain amount of your Qi, your vital energy, that which gives you life and makes you who you are, is inherited from your parents at birth. This portion of your body's composition is unalterable. But environment, diet, behavior, thought, and emotion also play an integral role in determining how healthy you will be. By leading a balanced life-style, you can maximize your ability to avoid disease and combat disease more successfully once it is manifest."

A system involving "pathogenic factors" opposed by "positive vitality" sounded very much like the Greek notion of "humors." According to the Greeks, there existed good and evil humors that, when balanced, resulted in the maintenance of health. The Greeks codified their theoretical system of humors around the same time Chinese scholars completed the *Yellow Emperor's Classic of Internal Medicine,* the fourth century B.C. In the West the humoral theory held sway until the eighteenth century. The Chinese system has far outlasted the Greek; twenty-four centuries after its inception it continues to influence the health practices of a billion people.

"Just how much illness is avoidable?" I asked Fang. "What types of illness can be influenced by our actions and our thoughts?"

"For us, these questions have been at the heart of medical theory for thousands of years," he replied. Once again he quoted from the medical treatise by the legendary Yellow Emperor: "I have heard that in early times the people lived to be over one hundred years old. Yet they remained active and did not become decrepit. These days, however, people reach only half that age and must curtail their activities. Does the world change from generation to generation, or does man become negligent of the laws of nature? Once there was temperance in eating and drinking. The hours of rising and retiring were regular and not disorderly or wild. By these means, those before us kept their bodies united with their souls to fulfill their allotted span, measuring up to one hundred years, before they passed away. Today people adopt recklessness as their usual behavior. They do not know how to find contentment within. They are not skilled in the control of their spirits. For these reasons, they reach only one-half of their one hundred years, and then they degenerate."

The notion that health depends on behavior and thought is a cornerstone of Chinese medical thought. To practitioners of traditional Chinese medicine, it is a certainty defined in terms of Yin and Yang and the concept of "Qi." To Western medical experts this same notion—that life-style and thought play a principal role in the determination of health and illness—remains an untested and controversial hypothesis.

The Qi Gong Masters

During the time of these early sessions with Fang and Old Chang, I began to hear rumors about the consummate mystics of China whose traditions, steeped in legend, involved the application of Chinese medical theory to physical feats of supernatural proportion. These mystics are called Qi Gong (chēē gōng) masters.

For traditional Chinese medicine, Qi is more than a concept; it is a physical reality. From a Western scientific standpoint, however, the existence of Qi is unproven. As a form of energy it remains unclassified. Its purported absence from the cadaver, in line with Chinese theory, makes postmortem research impossible. Acupuncture meridians, the conduits for Qi, are not identical to nerve routes or any other anatomical structures known to Western medicine. Efforts to analyze the Qi in anesthetized patients have failed because anesthesia supposedly relies on the disruption of Qi.

Qi Gong means "manipulation of vital energy," and the term refers to an ancient practice, crucial in the development of Chinese medicine. The masters of this practice, originally Daoist and Buddhist monks, are said to manipulate Qi within their bodies through special breathing exercises, physical training, and intense concentration. Qi Gong masters claim to control their Qi absolutely, directing it through any portion of their body at will in order to perform seemingly superhuman feats.

Between classes with Fang, I attended some popular performances. One bright, sunny day I sat in the audience of an acrobatic show in a park behind Beijing's Temple of Heaven. A bald Qi Gong master in his fifties, nude from the waist up, knelt on his hands and knees in front of a thick marble block. He stared at the block for several seconds, then began rocking back and forth on all fours. He breathed in sharply and deeply three times, tensed every muscle, let out a loud scream, and, using his forehead like a sledgehammer, split the marble block. The announcer raised his voice above the roar of the crowd to explain that the Qi Gong master had directed his Qi into his forehead in order to perform this feat.

At another performance, a Qi Gong master lay on a mat on a gymnasium floor while more mats were thrown over him. A dozen men carried a cement slab (supposedly weighing half a ton) onto the stage, positioned it over the Qi Gong master, and lowered it to his chest. Then they jumped onto the makeshift cement platform. The audience cheered. The men got down off the cement, removed it from the Qi Gong master's chest, and watched as he stood up—no thinner than he'd been before the act. The announcer told the audience that the Qi Gong master had directed his Qi into his upper body to keep from being crushed by the tremendous weight.

Another Qi Gong master directed his Qi into his hands and

used it to bend thick iron bars or smash boulders to bits. The next Qi Gong master claimed to place his Qi in the skin of his abdomen to balance the full weight of his body on top of a pitchfork. Quite unforgettable was the amazing Qi Gong master who used his Qi to "make his body hard as steel" and allowed a jeep to run over him.

Qi Gong masters inspire silence just by walking onstage. They are the embodiment of raw physical power tempered by serene monastic contemplation. At the climax of their act, whether it involves the shattering of stone or the suspending of a human body by an earlobe, a hush falls over the audience. Gasps are heard and then roars of applause. When the clapping dies down, a child may ask his father, "Papa, how did he do that? Did he really use his Qi? Did he, Papa?"

It's no wonder the Chinese people shower the remaining Qi Gong masters in China with adoration. During the 1960s, when they fell out of favor politically with the Gang of Four for being "superstitious and backward," Qi Gong masters nearly became extinct. Between 1964 and 1977 few people dared to practice or teach the art of Qi Gong in public. By 1979 a rebirth of this ancient practice was under way. Those few great Qi Gong masters still able to perform now resurfaced, attracting enormous crowds in parks and sports arenas and appearing on television and in magazines.

Were these performances merely circus acts carried off in grand tradition and style? I didn't pay much attention to the Qi Gong performances until a Chinese scientist friend asked whether I had seen the television documentary on Qi Gong. Apparently, the Shanghai Institute of Traditional Chinese Medicine, distinguished for its pioneering work on acupuncture analgesia, had recently begun scientific investigations of Qi Gong. The documentary, aired on national television, reviewed the history of Qi Gong, then made some startling claims. It suggested that Qi Gong masters had the ability not only to manipulate the Qi *within* their bodies but also to direct this Qi —in the form of energy—*outside* their bodies. The manipulation of Qi within the body was referred to as "internal Qi Gong"; the emission of Qi outside the body was called "external Qi Gong."

The television documentary had shown a Qi Gong master standing in front of an oscilloscope in a research laboratory. On command, the Qi Gong master huffed and puffed. He tensed his muscles to get his Qi flowing, directed it down his right arm, and then supposedly shot this Qi out his fingers. The oscilloscope registered little bleeps of energy each time the Qi Gong master fired away. The research laboratory had also taken pictures of what it said was Qi tracking down the extremities of Qi Gong masters, along the precise course of acupuncture meridians. The implications were that Qi existed as a physical force and that it could be emitted at will by Qi Gong masters.

Although I did not know it at the time, before long I would have a chance to investigate these strange phenomena face to face.

Tongues, Pulses, and Strange Diagnoses

It soon came time for Fang to prepare me for clinical work. According to traditional Chinese medicine, "Illness is comparable to the root. . . . If the root is not reached, the evil influences cannot be subjugated." Finding the "root" and detecting the nature of these "evil influences" are the objectives of traditional medical diagnosis. This diagnosis consists of "looking, listening, smelling, asking, and palpating"—without reflex hammers, blood pressure cuffs, or other Western tools.

The Tongue

Fang brought me to a small room at the Institute of Traditional Chinese Medicine where ten showcases held hundreds of life-sized replicas of human tongues (see photo). The artificial

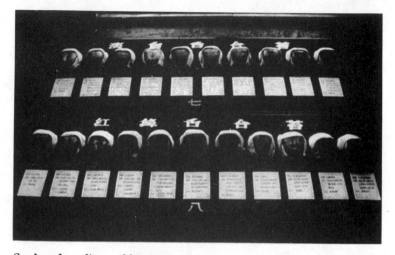

Sculpted replicas of human tongues—an educational tool in mastering Chinese medical diagnosis.

tongues displayed an astonishing variety of colors, textures, shapes, sizes, and coatings.

Traditional Chinese theory holds that the tongue is a sensitive daily barometer of human health. When illness strikes the body, the tongue changes dramatically, becoming yellow, swollen, cracked, or larded over with a thick mucous coating. To the experienced eye of a traditional doctor, these changes indicate specific bodily imbalances.

For example, a redder-than-normal tongue with a yellow, greasy coating corresponds to "excessive internal heat, dampness, and deficiency of bodily vital energy." A whiter-than-normal tongue with a thin coating reveals "a deficiency of Yang, vital energy, and blood." There are thousands of permutations and diagnostic combinations. A comprehensive medical education includes the study of hundreds of tongues.

Studying my own tongue, and those of the foreign doctors in

52

my dormitory, I could see how the tongue changes from day to day. On mornings when I awoke with a sore throat and swollen glands, my tongue became a deeper red and acquired a thick yellow coating. The possible relevance of the tongue's condition in the diagnosis of disease was even more apparent during my work in the medical clinics. Patients suffering from serious illness had tongues deviating from the normal color, texture, shape, and coating. Expert doctors of traditional medicine were able to predict the form of the tongue, without even seeing it, solely on the basis of the personal history given by the patient.

Specific bodily imbalances noted on physical examination of the tongue are clues to the "root" of the underlying medical problem. Chinese doctors use tongue diagnosis to direct their therapy and to follow the evolution of their patient's clinical condition.

Western physicians of the preantibiotic era paid attention to the appearance of the tongue but to a lesser extent than their Chinese counterparts. Today, Western doctors regard a tongue examination as a minor or insignificant aspect of a general physical examination. The West may be overlooking a highly valuable clinical tool—namely, the relationship between tongue morphology and specific physiological states.

The Pulse

Fang's lectures on tongue diagnosis were followed by a discussion of Chinese pulse taking. A traditional doctor feels for the pulse of the radial artery in the wrist. Western physicians touch the same area when they take a patient's pulse. However, they feel for only one pulse, whereas Chinese physicians feel for six pulses in each wrist: three superficial and three deep at specific points along the radial artery. Counting left and right, they find twelve pulses corresponding to twelve internal organs. The quality of each pulse reveals underlying imbalances in specific internal organs and in the body as a whole.

When ready to take the pulse, the traditional doctor taps two fingers on the examining table. Patients know they should hold out an upturned wrist for examination. The doctor places his or her left second, third, and fourth fingertips on the patient's right wrist. Then there is a pause, a moment of stillness and concentration.

Doctors study pulses for frequency, rhythm, strength, volume, and other characteristics. They use terms like *floating, slippery, bolstering-like, feeble, thready,* and *quick* to describe clinically the nature of the pulse. An abnormal pulse corresponds to a specific bodily imbalance. For example, a "superficial floating pulse," which is said to feel like "wood floating on water," indicates "external pathogenic factors" like excessive temperatures and commonly occurs in people with upper-respiratory infections.

The pulse, like the tongue, is a Chinese barometer of bodily function and dysfunction. Pulse taking requires years to master and is the traditional doctor's most important diagnostic skill. Fang maintained that by feeling the pulse one can accurately diagnose almost any medical problem.

Patient Interview

In addition to making tongue and pulse diagnoses, the traditional doctor inquires about the patient's complaints by recording what we in the West call a medical history. The objective of the history is to understand the patient's current complaints in detail.

The traditional doctor typically begins the interview with the question *"Ni you shenmo bing?"* Translated literally, this means "You have *what* illness?" but the phrase is taken to mean "What seems to be the problem?" The patient's response, known in Western terminology as the "chief complaint," is similar to that of patients in Western or traditional clinics: It's my headaches, It's this pain in my stomach, I've been feeling dizzy lately, and so on.

Thus far, the traditional doctor and his Western counterpart are on fairly common ground. But they soon diverge. Western-style doctors (the better ones, anyway) make a concerted effort to ask *open-ended* questions. An open-ended question cannot be answered with a simple yes or no and is meant to prod the patient into talking about the problem in his or her own words. For example, the question "What can you tell me about this discomfort?" is an open-ended one. "Did you also have pain in your back?" is a *directed* question; it requires a specific reply, yes or no. Traditional Chinese doctors make little use of open-ended questions and emphasize directed questioning.

Some of the questions asked by doctors of the two schools have no common ground at all. For example, traditional Chinese doctors pay extraordinary attention to changes in perspiration, appetite, and sensitivity to heat or cold. They regard the quality and duration of a fever, its association with a sense of coldness, and the coincident absence of perspiration or thirst as valuable clues in making a diagnosis. Western-style doctors ignore these details for the most part.

Diagnoses

Chinese medicine differs from its Western counterpart in its theoretical framework, its methods, and, most critically, its diagnoses—the labels of disease. A diagnosis made by a traditional

Chinese doctor bears no relation to a diagnosis uttered in any Western examinating room. For example, a case of pneumonia might carry the traditional Chinese diagnosis of "excess heat in the 'lung' and insufficient vital energy." Gastritis in an American doctor's office could be diagnosed as "extreme damp heat in the 'stomach' " in a Beijing examining room. *Pneumonia* and *gastritis* are Western words for specific human disorders. In China the same disorders are identified in an entirely different way.

According to Chinese medical theory, bodily dysfunction can be characterized in terms of "eight parameters." These include external versus internal, hot versus cold, excessive versus deficient, and Yin versus Yang. The first six are subservient to Yin and Yang, the theoretical foundation of Chinese medical practice.

A patient's symptoms and physical examination (tongue, pulse, etc.) enable the traditional doctor to recognize a pattern of illness in terms of "the eight parameters." This then becomes the *diagnosis*. Pneumonia might be called "an excess of heat in the 'lung' with a deficiency of Qi." Subsequent treatment with herbs or needles or diet would aim to correct this imbalance.

Imagine that you are a patient with pneumonia. You have a high fever, chills, and cough. When you arrive at the office of a Western doctor, a detailed medical history is taken and a physical examination and laboratory tests are performed. Evidence from your physical examination and abnormalities in your chest X ray lead the doctor to decide that you have pneumonia. A sample of your sputum, stained for bacteria, confirms the diagnosis. You are treated with appropriate antibiotics and sent home to rest in bed.

Now imagine going to the office of a traditional Chinese doctor with the same symptoms. The physician listens to your story and then asks a number of questions about the "type" of chills you've had and the manner of your sweating. He takes your pulse and examines your tongue. The doctor is aware that your lungs are troubling you, but his diagnosis, according to traditional medicine, refers to the underlying imbalances in your body. The pneumonia with its associated fever, cough, and sputum production is the *manifestation* of the underlying imbalance. It is the "uppermost branch," not the "root," of the illness. By studying your tongue and pulse and by listening to your story, the physician identifies the precise excess or deficiency affecting your body. This may involve an imbalance of an organ distant from the lung. The doctor treats your imbalance rather than a condition known as pneumonia.

Because traditional Chinese medical diagnoses frequently appear to have nothing in common with Western medical diagnoses, a comparison of the efficacy of Chinese and Western therapeutic techniques is extremely problematical.

For example, continue to imagine you have pneumonia. Once the Western physician has decided on a diagnosis of pneumococcal pneumonia, he prescribes an antibiotic known to be effective in eliminating the causative agent, which, according to Western medicine, is the pneumococcus. All patients diagnosed as having pneumococcal pneumonia are treated with the same antibiotic or class of antibiotics, and the clinical efficacy of these antibiotics can thereby be assessed.

A traditional doctor prescribes herbal remedies in a very different fashion. Let's imagine, for the sake of argument, that your tongue is redder than normal, a deep red at the tip, and has a yellow, greasy coating. This coating suggests a "damp heat" or "phlegm heat." The bright red tip of the tongue indicates "an excess of heat in the 'heart' or 'lung.' " Furthermore, if your pulse reveals any weakness of Qi, then you might expect to receive ten or twelve different herbs specifically to "reduce endogenous heat," "eliminate phlegm," and "strengthen vital energy." Just as penicillin is known in the West to kill pneumococcal pneumonia, so certain herbs are recognized in China to cool "heart" fires and "reduce endogenous heat." Traditional doctors prescribe these drugs on the basis not of the pneumococcal bacteria but of specific bodily imbalances that have led to a condition the Western doctor calls pneumococcal pneumonia.

This issue would be further confused if the herbal preparations were effective and Western researchers attempted to investigate their potency. For example, if your pneumonia responded dramatically within hours to a single combination of herbs, then the logical next step for a Western researcher might be to test these same herbs on fifty patients with documented pneumococcal pneumonia in order to arrive at a measure of effectiveness. According to traditional Chinese medicine, however, *each patient with symptoms is unique,* and each may have a different underlying imbalance causing the pneumonia. A traditional doctor might make fifty divergent diagnoses on our sample group of patients and then prescribe different combinations of herbs for each patient. In this situation, comparing the efficacy of one combination of herbs with that of antibiotics is like comparing apples with oranges.

Philosophically, the two schools follow different lines of scientific reasoning. The Western system proceeds along a line of a priori, cause-and-effect relations. The Chinese system employs a phenomenological, more circular logic. Both systems are internally consistent and capable of describing patterns of illness as well as methods of treatment. They are like two mathematical formulae applied to an identical problem. Both may work, but when placed side by side, the two models may nevertheless appear wholly unrelated.

The common element in Chinese and Western medicine is

chemistry—biochemistry. If the systems are both valid, they must both have the power to identify and change patterns in human chemistry. This is where the application of modern technology comes in. If the relations described by Yin and Yang, by the "five elements," and by the "eight parameters" are true, these relations must be capable of defining patterns of biochemistry—just as Western medicine does. If herbs and needles and changes in life-style are effective, they must be capable of predictably changing biochemical patterns. Traditional medical diagnoses and therapeutics must be standardized by means of Western methodology.

The two systems can be studied on a biochemical and pharmacological basis. In fact, much of this work is already in progress in and out of China. But there is a far simpler and more pragmatic approach to comparing these two systems. It requires no discussion of theory or biochemistry and no linear versus circular logic. It challenges the two systems to a duel. Since we do not know whether the Western or Chinese system is more effective in the treatment of lung cancer, for example, it might be beneficial to compare them in a controlled fashion. To do this we would treat half of a group of lung cancer patients with traditional medicine (herbs) and half with conventional Western chemotherapy. The functional outcomes of the two groups would then be compared. Theoretically, it should be possible to determine which approach, Western or Chinese, is more effective in altering the course of specific human illnesses.

Acupuncture: Unanswered Questions

In Western medical schools, after studying the preclinical sciences (such as biochemistry and microbiology), a student buys his first professional instruments: a stethoscope, an ophthalmoscope, a sphygmomanometer (blood pressure cuff), and other devices with Greek- or Latin-sounding names. This purchase is fraught with significance for the doctor-to-be. Although the tools are shiny bits of modern technology, the student handles them like sacred relics, making a silent prayer that some day he or she will know what the hell to do with them.

After two months of studying Chinese medical theory, I purchased my first Chinese medical instruments—acupuncture needles.

"Give me the best you've got," I told the saleswoman behind the counter of the Beijing Friendship Store. "My acupuncture class at the Institute of Chinese Medicine begins tomorrow, and

I want to have the finest needles available." My spoken Chinese was good, but my occasional literal translation of New York–ese made Chinese salesclerks laugh uncontrollably. The young woman behind the counter, her hair in long braids, her white blouse starched and buttoned to the collar, only half believed that I was a student at the Institute of Chinese Medicine. She opened the acupuncture display case, next to the baked goods and liquor, and showed me the finest needles in Beijing. I bought them all: long needles, short needles, plain needles, needles with fancy grips, needles on tiny hammers, needles specifically for ear lobes. I bought the books, the maps, and the posters of acupuncture meridians. I even bought the three-foot-high acupuncture doll with every acupuncture point and channel marked on its rubber surface—an educational Chinese voodoo doll.

"What will you do with all these needles?" said the saleswoman.

"I have no idea," I said, smiling back at her, "but I'll learn."

My acupuncture instructor was Dr. Zhang, director of the acupuncture clinic at the Dong Zhi Men Hospital. Zhang was in his forties and, like Fang, a native of northern China. He was tall and had awkwardly cut thick black hair. On the very top of his head the hairs stood straight up, but elsewhere they layered neatly to the sides. Zhang smiled a good deal but rarely laughed. A prominent vein running the length of his forehead filled to capacity in rare moments of excitement or anger. In general, though, Zhang was highly restrained. When it came to assessing acupuncture, he was slow to criticize and equally slow to boast of the efficacy of this ancient skill. He understood it, had lived it for twenty years, and was determined to show me what acupuncture could and could not accomplish. Zhang insisted I spend at least one month studying the theoretical basis of acupuncture before I entered any of the acupuncture clinics.

Zhang began my class with a discussion of "channels and collaterals." The channels, referred to as meridians, are distributed symmetrically over the human body. They are the road maps that enable one to locate specific acupuncture points. The channels are considered conduits for the flow of "blood" (血) and Qi (气) that connect internally with the viscera and externally with the skin and sense organs. There are twelve "major meridians," corresponding to twelve organs. In addition, there are eight "extra meridians" (known as collaterals) and a network of "minor meridians."* The channels interdigitate, so that the termination of one is the beginning of another. In this manner, acupuncture channels connect all portions of the human body. Weakness or illness in one area is said to influence other areas of the body via disruptions along the system of channels and collaterals.

This theory began with the discovery of key acupuncture points. The ancients believed that the stimulation of certain points on the surface of the body could relieve or cure diseases affecting the internal organs. They observed that sensations evoked by stimulation always traveled to other parts of the body along definite routes. By linking the acupuncture points of similar therapeutic effects along identical paths, they defined the system of channels and collaterals.†

Having made a diagnosis, the doctor carefully selects acupuncture points from the channel or channels most closely associated with the malady. For instance, if the underlying problem involves a primary heart ailment, then points along the heart

---

* Acupuncturists rely most heavily on the twelve major meridians and on two of the eight "extra meridians."
† There is recent archaeological evidence suggesting that the meridian theory predated the discovery of acupuncture points. See Wang Xue-tai, "Progress in Acupuncture Research," 1981.

meridian must be stimulated. The acupuncturist must choose "local points," that is, ones near the origin of the problem; "distant points," located far from the site of principal pathology; and, when appropriate, points known to reduce specific symptoms (cough, nausea, itching, etc.). Even though these points may be as far from one another as the forearm is from the calf, they are said to communicate in a predictable fashion via acupuncture channels.

The Points

The Chinese clinician uses acupuncture to diagnose illness. Studying relations between points on the skin and various internal organs, he learns to pay attention to tender or painful areas of the body. These sensitive areas, often referred to in the West as "trigger points," offer clues about the nature and location of the disease process.

Acupuncture can allegedly be used to *prevent* illness as well. By stimulating select acupuncture points, thereby adjusting channel and visceral function, a doctor may head off certain diseases—certain bodily imbalances—before they become problematical.

The stimulation of acupuncture points involves any of three methods: needle insertion, pressure, or heat. The needling procedure is called acupuncture. The use of finger pressure is Chinese massage (shiatsu is the Japanese equivalent). When heat is applied, usually in the form of slow-burning sticks of herbs (moxa),* the treatment is called moxibustion. When needles are used, they are twisted and/or connected to low-level electric generators for additional stimulation. These techniques all em-

---

* *Artemisia vulgaris,* also known as the Chinese mugwort.

ploy the same acupuncture points.

A Chinese medical student must memorize the twelve channels, fifteen collaterals, eight extra channels, and hundreds of acupuncture points defining these channels and collaterals. Dr. Zhang drilled me on the channels, their associations with one another, and their influence on the human body. He discussed acupuncture points in terms of exact location and indications for use. Puncturing a point was no easy task: size of needle, anatomical landmarks, and angle of insertion all had to be judged precisely. Every day, Dr. Zhang painted my body with dots at the acupuncture points to be discussed. Then he connected the dots with a marker to demonstrate the path of the channels. Body painting is a great teaching device. The problem was that Dr. Zhang painted with nearly indelible ink. Because the institute's hot water flowed only three or four times a week, I occasionally showed up at restaurants and United States embassy functions with my arms, legs, and head painted with stripes and dots.

After a couple of weeks of theory, I asked Dr. Zhang to let me practice with the needles. He insisted I go slowly: "Make small progress day by day." He suggested practicing acupuncture on inanimate objects before attempting to puncture flesh.

"It's surprising how difficult it is to insert a needle no thicker than a hair into something as tough and resistant as human skin," he said.

I practiced putting needles into cotton pin cushions, then graduated to layers of newspaper. Acupuncture needles are extremely delicate. I had a difficult time passing a needle through three sheets of newspaper without bending the needle. Dr. Zhang, on the other hand, could pass a needle half as thick as mine through thirty sheets of newspaper without bending it.

In order to perform acupuncture painlessly, one must insert

the needles quickly and smoothly without bending them.

"The skill is in the wrist," Zhang said. "If done correctly, there is no pain when entering the skin."

Before sticking others, I wished to be needled myself. Dr. Zhang said this wasn't necessary. But I wanted to understand the sensations involved, so that I could learn to elicit them properly in others. He warned me there might be some discomfort at first.

He was right.

He inserted a needle through a commonly used point between my right thumb and forefinger. It is called the *He Gu* point. On the first pass he went through the skin without causing any pain, but as he twisted the needle, he somehow harpooned a small nerve in my hand and sent a shock up my arm into my shoulder. I yanked my hand away, and held back a scream.

Dr. Zhang thought this was very funny: "You foreigners react this way at first. You are not used to the sensations of acupuncture."

Zhang stuck me again with the same needle in the same spot. This time there was no pain. Only after Zhang started to twist the needle to stimulate the point did I begin to feel a sensation of fullness, as if my hand were swelling from inside out. Then a feeling of distention went up my right arm into my upper back.

I asked Dr. Zhang whether patients always have some sort of sensation when they are needled. He told me that they should feel no pain associated with the piercing of the skin but that thereafter, when the point is stimulated, they will experience pain, soreness, heaviness, numbness, pins and needles, or the feeling of electric shock. Points on the face can cause a sensation of distention, while those on thick muscle tissue may feel sore. Pain is typical when patients are needled on thick-skinned body surfaces such as the palm, soles of the feet, and tips of the fingers or toes. A feeling of electric shock may be produced whenever true nerves along the body's extremities are disturbed.

The ancients had a specific name for the phenomena associated with these sensations. They called it *de Qi* (得气), which literally means "obtaining the Qi." Theoretically, needle insertion influences the flow of Qi (vital energy), which manifests itself in these altered sensations.

Each time the acupuncturist inserts a needle, he or she asks the patient, "Do you have it or not?" referring to the patient's having "obtained the Qi" or not. The question really asks whether the patient has felt a sensation of fullness, distention, pins and needles, or the like from the insertion of the needle in the spot being used. A reply of no means that the acupuncture point has not been stimulated and the acupuncturist has "missed." The needle is then removed and reinserted a few millimeters away or at a significantly different angle until the patient confirms that the phenomenon of *de Qi* has occurred.

Each time the attending physician had placed a needle in the foot of the hysterical "woman on the bus," he had asked whether she had "obtained the Qi." That peculiar interchange no longer mystified me.

Most Chinese have experienced acupuncture. They are not unduly frightened by it, and they understand the phenomenon of *de Qi*. In fact, the patient guides the acupuncturist by saying when an acupuncture needle has hit its mark and elicited the appropriate sensation.

By contrast, most Western patients seeking acupuncture therapy know nothing of the phenomenon of *de Qi*. Not knowing what sensations they should anticipate, they cannot tell the acupuncturist whether a needle is in the right place. When both therapist and patient know little about *de Qi*, as frequently occurs in Western acupuncture clinics, the result is bound to be disappointing.

Memorizing lists of acupuncture points and selecting them by way of some cookbook-style reference text (e.g., "for this symptom, puncture points A and B . . .") is not what acupuncture is about. A Chinese acupuncturist spends years as an apprentice learning to diagnose and treat ill patients and to recognize their response to acupuncture needling and the phenomenon of *de Qi*. To become an acupuncturist in China today one must complete a rigorous education in traditional Chinese medicine and then specialize in acupuncture. This takes as long as it does to become a licensed surgeon in the West—about six or seven years.

Needle insertion is said to be most therapeutic when the sensations are noticeable, instantaneous, and conducted a good distance away from the acupuncture point. The intensity of the sensations typically varies with the physical condition of the patient. Acutely ill patients usually have more intense sensations and tend to refer sensations to more distant body parts. The theoretical reason for this is that sicker patients have greater excesses or deficiencies of Qi. Thus, any correction of these imbalances by acupuncture will be more noticeable for the patient.

The great controversy among Chinese acupuncturists is whether Qi has a physical reality that the practitioner can sense and alter. Acupuncturists of the old school insist they can "feel" the Qi through the needle in their fingers when they have entered the appropriate point or channel. A Chinese maxim holds, "When the Qi is obtained, it is like a fish that has taken the bait." Some acupuncturists also contend, quite heatedly, that they can not only *sense* Qi but also *transmit* it through the acupuncture needle to the appropriate point in the patient's body.

The controversy gains drama from acupuncture's use in surgery for anesthesia or analgesia. Acupuncture clearly does well as a substitute for Western drugs, but how it does so remains frustratingly unclear.

Acupuncture Analgesia

One surgical operation convinced me that acupuncture analgesia can dramatically alter human physiology. I was invited to the Beijing Neurosurgical Institute to assist in a major surgical operation performed under acupuncture analgesia. Chinese medical publications have recently stopped referring to acupuncture "anesthesia," or absence of sensation; instead, they now talk of acupuncture "analgesia," or pain relief.

A fifty-eight-year-old Beijing University professor of history named Lu had a brain tumor. Lu had been in excellent health, but at fifty-six he developed problems with his vision and simultaneouly noted some dizziness and loss of libido. He was eventually referred to the Beijing Neurosurgical Institute, where an X ray of his skull revealed a chestnut-size growth located in the center of his brain. The growth was probably a benign tumor originating from his pituitary gland. This type of tumor could explain all of Professor Lu's symptoms. If it was removed and proven to be benign, Lu could lead a healthy and symptom-free existence. The problem was how to remove such a sizable growth.

When a pituitary tumor is discovered early, a surgeon gets at it through the patient's nose. Lu's tumor was too big for this procedure. It had to be approached from the top of his skull, and that meant cutting through a bony portion of the cranium.

Lu's neurosurgeon, Dr. Wang Zhong-cheng, suggested he have the procedure done under acupuncture analgesia as opposed to conventional anesthesia. At first, Dr. Wang told me, Lu was not too enthusiastic about the idea. He had only limited exposure to acupuncture and was not a devout proponent of traditional Chinese medicine. He was also understandably unnerved by the prospect of being totally awake and responsive during brain surgery. However, after Dr. Wang told him that more than 90 percent of all head and neck surgeries at the Neurosurgical Institute were performed successfully under acupuncture analgesia and that acupuncture had significantly fewer side effects than other forms of anesthesia, Professor Lu agreed to give it a try. Conventional Western-style anesthesia would be available in the operating room and could be used at a moment's notice if necessary. I watched the surgery and assisted with the acupuncture.

I scrubbed and gowned just as I would have in a Western operating room, except that my gown was made of reusable cotton rather than disposable paper. When I entered the operating amphitheater, Comrade Lu was stretched out on the operating table. He was alert and quite willing to talk to a foreign guest.

The operating room was old and clean. There was no shiny, high-tech equipment to speak of. Countless cleanings had left the tile walls a spotless white, without luster. The IV tubing was of reusable rubber, the IV bottle refillable. The high-intensity lamp used as the spotlight for the surgery took up most of the ceiling. It was an archaic but impressive mass of incandescent bulbs and polished, curved mirrors. Professor Lu lay on his back on an immobile operating table below the lights. His head was clean-shaven. He wore plaid pajamas and was already covered from the neck down by layers of white surgical sheets.

A woman dressed in surgical attire entered the operating room with a brisk, confident stride. She sat on the stool next to the operating table, paused with her hands in her lap, and studied the equipment in the room. She then introduced herself as one of the staff anesthesiologists. This woman was thoroughly trained in both Chinese and Western medicine. She had practiced conventional Western anesthesia for ten years before she first touched an acupuncture needle, in the 1950s. For twenty years she had been part of a special research team responsible for integrating acupuncture with surgical anesthesia. Head and neck procedures were her specialty. She carried a well-worn stethoscope in one pocket and five sets of acupuncture needles in the other.

Next to the operating table was the familiar fire-engine-red "crash cart." It held the standard Western anesthetic agents to be used for a "crash"—a speedy induction of anesthesia if the acupuncture failed.

Lu had an intravenous line in place and through it received a mild preoperative sedative consisting of 0.1 mg of fentanyl (a narcotic) and 5.0 mg of haloperidol (a sedative/antipsychotic drug). These medications would relax and sedate the patient, but they would not provide adequate anesthesia.

The next step was the insertion of needles and the beginning of acupuncture stimulation. The anesthesiologist selected six key points on the basis of the collective experience of the team of doctors in hundreds of similar operations.

The first two points were in the region of the eyebrows—one in the middle of the left eyebrow, the other at the inner (medial) aspect of the right eyebrow (the part closest to the bridge of the nose). The anesthesiologist inserted a single needle, six inches long, into the left eyebrow and directed it under the skin across the bridge of the nose into the area of the right-eyebrow point. The needle did not exit the skin but merely traversed the region between the eyebrows starting and ending at the pair of acupuncture points. The needle was then twisted by hand for initial stimulation until Comrade Lu "obtained the Qi"—that is, ex-

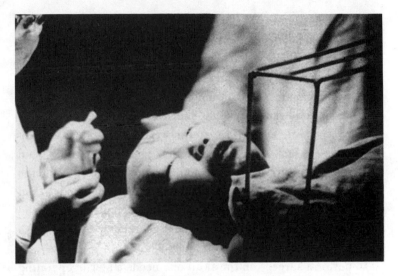

Acupuncture analgesia for brain surgery.

perienced a sensation of fullness, distention, and mild electric shock at both points.

The anesthesiologist then attached a low-voltage electric stimulator to the protruding end of the needle in order to send electric current through it at fixed intervals. The frequency of stimulation was easily observable in the slight twitch of the facial muscles in the area. In the same manner with the same kinds of equipment, she stimulated two other points near the right temple. Once again, Comrade Lu reported a feeling of fullness when these needles were stimulated by hand or electricity.

The final two points to be stimulated were in the region of the left shin and ankle. The anesthesiologist used separate needles for these points and connected two more electronic stimulators, by way of wires leading to a heavy black metal box about the size of a car battery. The device was, in fact, nothing more than a twelve-volt battery that could deliver current at specific frequencies. The battery sat on the floor next to the operating table. The four sets of wires attached to needles in Lu's forehead and left lower extremity were connected to the battery stimulator. As the machine was turned up and the amperage increased, Lu's calf and brow began to twitch ever so slightly.

"De Qi le mei you?" ("Do you have the Qi?"), the anesthesiologist asked Lu. *"De le, De le* ("I have it, I have it still"), said Lu. Then came an induction period of twenty minutes. While the surgeons arranged their equipment, the anesthesiologist asked me to take the patient's initial temperature, pulse, and blood pressure—his vital signs. Lu and his surgeons waited for the acupuncture analgesia to take effect.

To perform surgery on the skull one needs a sterile operating field and some mechanical assurance that the patient's head is not going to move during the procedure. This latter requirement is of special importance when an *alert* patient undergoes brain surgery. A specially designed metal halo frame was used to secure Lu's head in place and to serve as a scaffold for sterile drapes. The frame was made from four metal rods. Three were straight, and the fourth had a half-moon, padded metal band at its center. This "halo" fitted over Lu's forehead and bolted to the operating table. The three remaining sides of the frame formed an empty rectangular space over Lu's face. From the top of the frame sterile sheets descended like a curtain over Lu's forehead. Using this arrangement, one could keep the top of Lu's skull sterile while his face and body remained uncovered. Lu could see and talk to the anesthesiologist and me, but he could not see the surgeons at work.

The doctors encouraged me to chat with Lu. They gave me a seat next to the operating table so that I could monitor his pulse and blood pressure while talking with him during the procedure.

Since pulse rates and blood pressure rise with the onset of pain, it would be critical for me to follow these parameters during the procedure. Apart from the small preoperative doses of sedatives and narcotics (5.0 mg of haloperidol and 0.1 mg of fentanyl), there was no further pharmacological sedation or analgesia during the surgical procedure. The patient's pain relief came exclusively from acupuncture.

The chief surgeon took a marking pen and outlined the four-by-six-inch rectangle of bone charted for removal from the left side of Lu's skull. Then he took a pin and jabbed the skin of this rectangular area. Lu said he felt slight pressure, but no pain. The surgeons and the anesthesiologist, pleased with the degree of anesthesia, cleansed and prepared the site of incision.

As I took a reading of Lu's vital signs and began a conversation with him, he was a bit groggy from preoperative medications. Aside from feeling sleepy, he was fine. He moved his fingers and toes without difficulty, and his speech was clear.

The anesthesiologist gave the go-ahead to begin, and the surgeons took up their scapels. They made an incision along three sides of the rectangle outlined by the marking pen, and proceeded to lift a three-sided flap of full-thickness skin from Lu's skull. At the moment of incision, Lu failed to wince, grimace, or give any hint of pain. He remarked that he was aware of the surgeons applying pressure to his skin but that he experienced no discomfort. His pulse and blood pressure remained at their preoperative levels.

Using high-speed bone drills with surgical bits, the surgeons bored holes through the four corners of the rectangular piece of bone. They threaded a wire saw between two adjacent holes and pulled it back and forth until the bone was sawed through. They repeated this procedure on all four sides of the rectangle until they could remove the large piece of bone. The manipulation of bony surfaces is usually extremely painful.

Lu said he felt no pain. His pulse and blood pressure remained unchanged. I asked him what was "on his mind." He laughed and said he was wondering whether Americans ever used acupuncture analgesia in their operations. He was calm, responsive, and talkative as surgeons removed pieces of his skull while a few, well-placed needles protected him from pain.

Throughout the entire procedure, which continued for more than four hours, Lu remained conscious, and his vital signs remained stable. We conversed the whole time he was on the operating table.

After the completion of the surgery, Lu sat up from the operating table, shook the hand of his surgeon, thanked him profusely, shook hands with the anesthesiologist and me, then walked out of the operating room unassisted. The large tumor had been successfully removed, and it subsequently proved to be benign.

Some weeks later I participated in two thyroid operations done at the Dong Zhi Men Hospital. In certain respects these neck operations performed under acupuncture analgesia were even more impressive than Professor Lu's brain surgery. A thyroidectomy (surgical removal of the thyroid gland) requires an extensive dissection of the neck and is almost always performed with the patient under general anesthesia. In the thyroid operations using acupuncture analgesia, no drugs whatsoever were administered. The analgesia consisted of two needles in the hand and nothing else. During this operation, too, the patient remained alert and comfortable, the vital signs remained stable, and the clinical results were most impressive.

Although acupuncture has existed for more than three thousand years, its application as a surgical analgesic is barely twenty-five years old. Surgery played a minor role in the evolu-

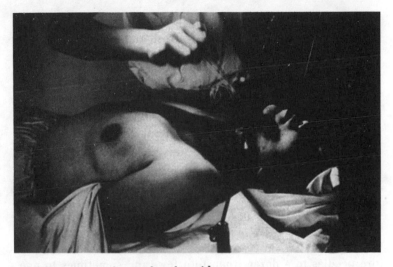

Acupuncture analgesia for thyroid surgery.

tion of traditional Chinese medicine. This was due in part to the Confucian concept of filial piety, which views the body as the ultimate gift of one's parents and surgery as a mutilation of that gift. Herbal remedies and acupuncture were consequently considered superior to surgery. Traditional Chinese doctors performed minor surgical procedures, such as the suturing of wounds, but they rarely attempted major surgery.*

It was not until the 1950s, when Chairman Mao called for the union of Chinese and Western medicine, that acupuncture was applied to major surgery. Chinese researchers postulated that acupuncture, which had successfully controlled pain in a variety of conditions, could be performed on patients just prior to major surgery and thereby be used to reduce the amount of anesthetic

---

* A notable exception was the famous traditional physician Hua Tuo, who used herbal anesthetic prescriptions while attempting abdominal and brain surgery in the third century A.D.

medication required. The theory proved correct, and acupuncture analgesia was born in surgical research laboratories in the late 1950s.

The first successful application of acupuncture analgesia involved a thoracotomy (open-chest surgery), performed in Liuzhou in 1957. Tonsillectomies done under acupuncture analgesia were performed in Shanghai and Xian in 1958. Medical researchers soon applied the new technique to all areas of surgical exploration. Initially, an intra-abdominal or an open-chest operation required the simultaneous skills of four or five acupuncturists inserting over one hundred needles. By experimenting on themselves to determine the degree of analgesia, medical researchers reduced the number of necessary acupuncture needles to a dozen, then to a few, and sometimes to one.

In the 1960s and 1970s Chinese anesthesiologists and surgeons experimented extensively with acupuncture anesthesia and its application to a variety of surgical procedures. Head and neck, abdominal, gynecological, and thoracic (heart and lung) surgery was performed under acupuncture anesthesia. With experience, problems surfaced. Although success rates in head and neck surgeries under acupuncture analgesia were greater than 90 to 95 percent, acupuncture failed to give adequate pain relief in 20 to 30 percent of all abdominal, gynecological, or chest surgery.*

Unlike conventional anesthesia, acupuncture analgesia failed both to relax the abdominal muscles (an important aspect of

---

* This information was provided by the Department of Anesthesia, Beijing Neurosurgical Institute, and the Beijing Institute of Traditional Chinese Medicine. See also Joseph Needham's May 1977 lecture to the Medical Acupuncture Society, printed in Alexander Macdonald, *Acupuncture: From Ancient Art to Modern Medicine* (London: George Allen & Unwin, 1982), 121.

abdominal surgery) and to block pain associated with the stretching of internal organs (these pain fibers are controlled by the vagus nerve). By the 1980s Chinese departments of anesthesia were employing acupuncture primarily for head and neck procedures, but not for abdominal, gynecological, or thoracic operations.

Acupuncture analgesia works, in certain cases, but no one knows precisely why it works. Over the past few years scientists have discovered that acupuncture stimulates the production of certain morphine-like substances in the brain. These substances diminish pain perception. The newly discovered compounds are called endorphins or enkephalins. They are small chains of amino acids that serve as neuromodulators, that is, regulators of neurological activity. There is evidence that acupuncture influences the production and distribution of a great many neuromodulators and neurotransmitters and that this in turn alters the perception of pain.

Not all patients respond well to acupuncture analgesia, however. Is success due to a patient's genetic makeup, say, an excess or deficiency of certain enzymes? Or does it depend on his or her belief system, on an acceptance that acupuncture will in fact relieve pain? How much does success or failure depend on the skill of the acupuncturist? Do those who show a marked response to acupuncture needles tend to be highly suggestible? The Shanghai Acupuncture Research Unit has used acupuncture analgesia on animals, so it is unlikely that belief systems and suggestibility are solely responsible for the entire phenomenon.* On the other hand, there is growing evidence that psychological factors may significantly alter a given patient's physio-

---

* See also Evert Lagerweij et al., "The Twitch in Horses: A Variant of Acupuncture," *Science* 225 (1984): 1172–74.

logical response to acupuncture. There seems to be a combined effect involving psychology and physiology in acupuncture, and the Chinese are studying this question in greater depth.

Second Encounter:
The Sisters Wang

On March 11, 1979, the *Sichuan Daily* ran a curious story about a twelve-year-old boy named Tang Yu. Allegedly, Tang Yu "read words with his ears." He could "read" whatever was written on a piece of paper simply by holding the paper to his ear. Tang Yu's talents were referred to as "exceptional human body functions," and news of his "discovery" spread quickly throughout China.

Within months newspapers from other provinces carried stories about similar psychic abilities of dozens of school-age children. Most striking were accounts of two sisters from Beijing—the Wang sisters.

It was said that if you gave them any kind of box and put a piece of paper in the box, they could—merely by touching the box—tell you in accurate detail what was written on the paper. They could even tell you the color of ink used. The children claimed to "see" the written contents of the message inside the container. Even stranger was their claim that if one sister got the box containing a written word, she could communicate this thought to the other by telepathy. Rumor held that these children could even see the outline of internal organs simply by looking at a patient's body; that they could see large tumors or collections of fluid anywhere in the body; that they could see a heart beating and tell a physician precisely how fast it was beating; and that they could determine the hair length and sex of an unborn fetus by inspecting the abdomen of a pregnant woman.

I asked my teachers at the Institute of Traditional Chinese Medicine whether they knew of the Wang sisters. My instructors had not only heard of them, but had actually tested them. The two children had visited the Institute of Medicine and had thoroughly convinced the medical faculty of their psychic power. The tests had been repeated many times, and the faculty believed in the sisters.

I had not learned of these unique investigations, because the whole topic remained a sensitive area of Chinese research. It was a kind of state secret.

Though skeptical myself, I wanted very much to meet these girls. After overcoming miles of bureaucratic red tape, a friend of a friend arranged a group visit to the Wang sisters' home. Twelve Chinese doctors trained in Western medicine, most of them surgeons and all of them great skeptics, formed the rest of the party.

Our bus pulled up in front of a small lane in the northwest corner of Beijing. Tiny, one-story brick homes lined the lane and adjacent alleyways. The makeshift roofs were of corrugated metal, wood, and tarpaulin. It was a hot summer day, doors were open, and I could see into all the cramped little rooms that served as kitchen, bedroom, and dining room for entire families. Long ropes and bamboo poles draped with laundry connected one house to the next. Halfway down the alley was the familiar public toilet—a functional gray concrete-and-plaster outhouse with holes in the ground. Trees dotted the beginning and end of the lane, but the ground around the houses was unpaved dirt. In the middle of the dusty alley, a hunchbacked old man sat on a wicker chair, smoking a pipe and listening to a radio broadcast of Beijing opera music.

As we approached the narrow dirt path leading to the Wang home, dozens of neighbors filed out to see what was going on. The word *wai guo ren* (foreigner) ricocheted from one end of the lane to the other. By this time (May of 1980) these people were accustomed to the sight of large delegations of native scientists parading down their alleyway. The Wang sisters had, after all, been under investigation for months. However, there had been few, if any, foreign visitors in this Beijing neighborhood.

Mr. Wang met our group at the doorstep. He extended his hand to me, grasped my forearm, and smiled warmly. He turned his head to one of the surgeons, obviously thinking he had to use an interpreter.

"Please tell this foreign friend that he is a welcome guest."

I clasped Mr. Wang's hand and in my best Chinese said, "I have looked forward to meeting you and your children for some time. My deepest thanks to you and your wife for allowing this visit."

Mrs. Wang giggled in the doorway, "Oh, you can speak Mandarin, how wonderful!"

Mrs. Wang pointed at two children jumping rope in front of a tree at the side of the lane.

81

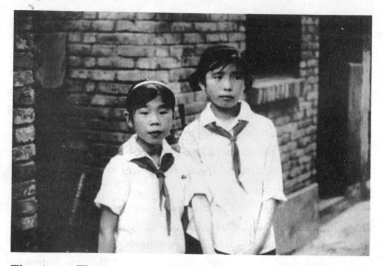

The sisters Wang—exceptional human body functions?

"Those are my daughters whom you have come to see. The little one, Wang Bin, is eleven, and the big one, Wang Qiang, is thirteen."

So these were the remarkable sisters Wang. They appeared no different from other Chinese children. Each wore a white blouse and a patriotic red scarf around her neck. The two jumped rope in the traditional way, with a long, multicolored string of rubber bands stretched around a tree and the calves of one sister while the other jumped in and out of the loop. They giggled like their mother, chewed gum, and kept a polite distance from the grown-ups.

"Come meet these doctors and our American friend," Mrs. Wang called to the girls.

The girls stepped out of their jump rope, ran toward us, looked first at their parents for approval, and then without even a trace of shyness said informally, "Hello, Dr. Ai Sen Bo.

What have you got for us to read?"

Mrs. Wang suggested we first go inside for tea.

We walked through a small room that served as entrance, kitchen, and dining room, then into a second small room, which was the sleeping quarters for the Wang family. Family and visitors together, eighteen people sat elbow to elbow on the two beds, a desk, and a tiny end table lining the periphery of the room. The two Wang sisters brought in wooden stools and sat in the center of our circle. Mrs. Wang served tea as she and her husband shared a little family history.

"We are factory workers, Mr. Wang and I, and our family is one of the Old Hundred Surnames," said Mrs. Wang. This was her way of telling us they were common people without special status or Party affiliation. There were four Wang children, but only the second and third displayed any special abilities. In school the girls had no better than an average record.

The sisters asked whether we had prepared anything for them.

I took a black plastic film container from my pocket. I had previously inserted a tiny piece of folded paper with two Chinese characters written on it. The characters were 朋友 (pronounced "peng you" and meaning "friend"). I handed the container to the older sister.

At the same time, one of the surgeons produced his own container constructed from thick black protective jackets used to insulate X-ray film. He had sandwiched a piece of paper with the word 人 (pronounced "ren" and meaning "man") between sheets of this opaque paper. The sandwich was sealed with adhesive tape. The younger sister took this container.

No one but the authors themselves knew what was written on the papers in these containers.

The two girls sat cross-legged on the stools, bouncing one leg

atop the other and chewing gum incessantly. I was on the edge
of my seat. The neurosurgeons leaned back smugly and crossed
their arms across their chests.

Each girl wrapped her left fist around her container and then
jammed the fist under her right armpit. Mrs. Wang explained it
wasn't necessary for the containers to be placed under the armpit, but it was important for the girls to have skin contact to
"read" the contents. Apparently, they had by experiment found
the right armpit to be the most functional body site.

I joked that I might have written my words in English. The
younger sister said, smiling, that we could write in any language
or draw simple pictures if we wished. She could reproduce
whatever was on the paper even if she didn't understand its
meaning. It would take anywhere from a few seconds to fifteen
minutes for the written contents to "materialize."

The girls explained that the characters (or pictures) actually
became visible to them "as if appearing on a screen on the inside
of [their] foreheads." They didn't know how or why this happened. They told us this "screen" was small, and that if the
characters given them were more than an inch high on the paper,
then the "picture" might not fit onto the inside of their foreheads.

We asked Mrs. Wang how her daughters' marvelous talents
had been discovered. She told us that months prior to our visit
Mr. Wang had been reading the newspaper story about Tang Yu,
the little boy from Sichuan who could "read" without seeing.
Over the dinner table, the children admitted they had also had
this sensation and been surprised that their father considered
this unique. In fact, they had assumed everyone could do this
to some extent. From that day forward, the parents began investigating the girls' abilities in greater depth with the help of local
researchers.

It sounded impressive. Nonetheless, it was hard to believe.

The big sister, still holding my canister with the words *peng you* under her armpit, blurted out, *"Peng, peng, peng you!!!"*

I was amazed. I had written those words in my own room, twenty miles away fifteen hours earlier, and shown them to no one.

The little sister took the gum out of her mouth just long enough to say, *"Ren!* My word is *ren!* And you wrote it in red ink!"

They repeated this stunt seven times, as we all took turns going hundreds of yards from the house to scribble tiny words or pictures onto small pieces of paper, which we then sealed in boxes.

They got six out of seven *exactly* correct.

Their only error was a curious one. I had gone outside with my film canister and small pieces of blank paper. I wrote 中国 (*Zhong Guo,* China). But then I decided that 中国 was too simple. I ripped up that piece of paper, took out another, and wrote 美国 (*Mei Guo,* America). I folded the paper four times, placed it in the film container, returned to the Wang bedroom, and handed it to the big sister. She read it as *Zhong Guo.* Was it possible that the writing within the container was less important than the mental image projected by the person who wrote it? My initial, perhaps stronger, thought was *Zhong Guo.* I should have devised a more appropriate experiment. I should have written a word, placed it in the container, and asked a friend to hand it to the children. In this way the author would have been absent when the girls attempted the reading.

In spite of their single failure, about which they were quite embarrassed, the girls' numerous accurate successes transformed every physician in the room into a believer. Before leaving, we saw one last demonstration.

I wrote down the character for *fire*— 火, "huo"—and shoved the paper into the container. Big sister promptly placed it under her armpit. Then I turned to little sister and said, "Okay, without your sister saying a word, tell me what's on the paper." She smiled, chewed her gum, stared at her sneakers, and waited for big sister to get her brain waves oscillating. In about two minutes, big sister said, "I know what the word . . ." Little sister interrupted, shouting out, *"Ren! I see ren!"* The character *ren* — 人 (man)—is just two tiny slashes from 火 (*huo,* meaning "fire"). I told the little sister that she was incorrect and needed to try harder. Her eyeballs turned upward as she concentrated on her forehead in an animated trance.

"It's like *ren,*" she said, "only a little different. I'll draw for you what I see, but it doesn't make any sense."

She wrote 仌, which has no meaning in the Chinese language. However, because what she wrote was so close to my original character, though not exactly correct, it seemed more possible than ever that she indeed visualized the containers' contents— or, more probably, my mental image—and faked nothing.

The neurosurgeons were also humbled. "I would never have believed this without seeing it with my own eyes," remarked a senior surgeon. He quoted the *Book of Changes:* "I am reminded that haughtiness invites ruin; humility receives benefits."

The Wang sisters were pleased that they had convinced us. They were also glad to meet a real, live American. I wanted to spend more time with them, and they obliged with a kind invitation to go boating the next week.

A few days later, however, I heard through the grapevine that certain "official channels" were upset that "unofficial channels" had been used to arrange my meeting with the Wang sisters. For me to see them again, unofficially, might be risky for them or for my friends who had made the introduction as a personal favor.

I never saw these magical children again.

Doctors of traditional medicine were not as amazed by the Wang sisters as the doctors of Western medicine who visited them with me. Skills identical to those of the Wang sisters had been observed among masters of traditional medicine for centuries and were documented in historical texts. Telepathy, clairvoyance, and psychokinesis were part of the Chinese medical tradition.

In February 1980 the popular magazine *Ziran Zazhi* (Nature) sponsored a national conference on parapsychology in Shanghai. That spring millions of people crammed into sports arenas to watch Qi Gong masters perform incredible feats. Explanations in the popular press for the "exceptional human body functions" noted both in children and in Qi Gong masters came from ancient *medical* literature. This connection fascinated me, and I decided to find a medical expert who could clarify these anomalous phenomena.

My instructors in the acupuncture and herbal-medicine clinics suggested I meet with Dr. Ren Ying-qiu, one of China's foremost scholars of traditional medicine. Dr. Ren, then a senior professor at the Beijing Institute of Traditional Chinese Medicine, had practiced clinical medicine for fifty years and written hundreds of papers on the technique and theory of traditional medicine.

We met in Dr. Ren's tiny study on the third floor of an urban high rise. Books on medicine and philosophy lined the room. A calligraphy painting with a quotation from the *Yellow Emperor's Classic of Internal Medicine* hung above Ren's desk. The office smelled like a musty, subterranean rare-book library.

Dr. Ren, a man in his seventies, leaned back in his reclining chair, lit a filterless cigarette, and glanced toward the doorway as I entered. A woolen cap covered his balding head; his feet barely touched the floor from the chair. His face was badly wrinkled, blemished with brown old-age spots. His dark eyes had pored over countless books, scrutinized the illnesses of thousands of patients, and examined the weight of evidence supporting the efficacy of traditional medicine. Ren pushed aside his quill pen and reached for his ashtray, overflowing with crumpled butts. He took long puffs on his cigarette between sentences.

"Welcome, welcome," he said, while getting up from his chair.

"I have heard much about you, Dr. Ai. I have been told you are interested in the integration of Chinese and Western medicine. Is this the nature of your visit to China?"

"Yes, this is why I have come," I said.

"Where did you learn to speak Mandarin?"

"I studied Chinese at Harvard University. My teachers were originally from Beijing."

"You're studying Chinese medicine at the institute now, are you not?"

"Yes."

"In what way can I help you?"

"I've come here to get your opinion about the nature of Qi. I've heard reports about gifted children and Qi Gong masters performing all sorts of feats including telepathy and the emission of energy at will. Have you had experience with this sort of activity?"

"Yes, I have. Between your words you are saying that you do not believe in Qi Gong. Is that right?"

"I don't know what to believe about Qi," I answered. "If it exists, then it has not been identified by Western medical science."

"Have you observed acupuncture analgesia?"

"Yes."

"Do you believe that this is effective?"

"Yes, I do."

"Well, acupuncture depends entirely on the flow of Qi. The acupuncturist senses and directs Qi through the needle. Acupuncture without Qi is only as effective as one man's sticking needles into the flesh of another. This would serve no purpose. Chinese massage is the same. Qi can be used to heal in many situations. It has been used therapeutically for thousands of years and is basic to all of Chinese medicine. Let me assure you, it is a physical reality."

"What about the claims that it is possible to direct Qi within the body and emit it externally? What about telepathy and psychokinesis? Are these claims true?"

"They are all true, Dr. Ai. Throughout recorded history, Qi Gong masters, who were also the consummate physicians, performed wondrous tasks that might seem inexplicable to you. For example, during the period of the Warring States [403–221 B.C.], the historian Si Ma-qian recounted the sensational abilities of Bian Que, a man reportedly able to see through opaque objects. In the age of the Three Kingdoms [220–264 A.D.] the famous physician Hua Tuo.displayed talents identical to those of the Wang sisters and the Qi Gong masters currently performing throughout China. All these skills can be explained in terms of the manipulation of Qi. In the rare child, perhaps one in a million, these exceptional human body functions are inborn, but without appropriate exercises they will diminish and disappear. The practice of Qi Gong techniques will induce these exceptional human body functions, and Qi Gong can be learned by anyone. I have experienced these things myself, and I am convinced they are not false words."

"You are the first American medical exchange student to study traditional medicine in the People's Republic of China. If you are to accomplish your objective, then you must be convinced of the existence of Qi. Without Qi there is no Chinese medicine. Without an understanding of Qi, Western medicine, with all its powerful science, will remain ignorant of the single greatest gift of Chinese medicine. It is real, this Qi, and you should make every effort while you are in China to study it— to be convinced of its significance."

Other senior faculty at the Institute of Traditional Chinese Medicine echoed Dr. Ren's advice. These were men of incomparable reputation. Their belief in the existence of Qi and the significance of Qi Gong was unwavering. Later they would introduce me to a real Qi Gong master.

In the Clinic:
Acupuncture
and Massage

For three months, I worked in the acupuncture clinic of the Dong Zhi Men Hospital with Dr. Zhang. Dong Zhi Men is one of the four major Beijing hospitals devoted exclusively to traditional Chinese medicine. Dr. Zhang and I saw approximately 100 patients a day. The outpatient department as a whole, which included the herbal-medicine and massage clinics in addition to the acupuncture clinic, treated between 1,500 and 2,000 patients a day. This is roughly ten times the number of patients seen in the outpatient department of most American hospitals.

Who were all these people and how were they referred? The answer is not simple. We know a good deal about the delivery of Western-style medical practice in China. We know very little, however, about the referral patterns of patients seeking traditional medical care. In 1980 there were 502,000 Chinese doctors trained in Western medicine, as well as 369,000 practicing doctors of traditional Chinese medicine.* Not everyone was going to a Western-style doctor for his or her care.

The referral system for Western medical practice is as follows. A patient must be referred from a local street hospital or factory hospital to a district hospital, and then, if necessary, to a municipal or specialty hospital. In the rural areas, where more than 800 million people live, the referral pattern involves barefoot doctors, brigade health stations, commune clinics or hospitals, and ultimately county hospitals. The county, municipal, and specialty hospitals serve as teaching and research centers throughout China. But these are by and large Western medical facilities.

How tens of millions of patients get to acupuncture and massage clinics is not altogether clear. The manner of their referral to Western-style hospitals from traditional clinics remains a mystery. Patients have the choice of Western or traditional Chinese medicine. Although no statistics are available, it is probably safe to say that the older and more rural populations prefer traditional medicine to Western medicine, whereas the younger, more urban, and better-educated populations prefer Western medicine. And after more than a century's exposure to both systems of medicine, people have developed treatment preferences for particular types of illness. In general, they feel that chronic illness and musculoskeletal problems are more amenable to traditional techniques but that acute problems like trauma or overwhelming infections are best treated with Western techniques. These are generalizations, however, because both systems of medicine claim to be effective for most medical problems. Some patients are fickle and go back and forth be-

* Ministry of Public Health Statistics, 1980.

tween Western and traditional medical clinics. Others, fed up with one style of medicine, select the other by default.

In the hallway outside the room where Dr. Zhang and I worked, hundreds of patients stood in the entryway or sat on long wooden benches waiting for their number to be called. They had obtained numbered tickets after paying a fee on entry to the clinic. The fee was five or ten fen, or roughly two or three dollars in terms of Western income. There were no prescheduled appointments, no secretaries, no phones, no computer terminals. Everyone took a number and waited.

All Chinese patients carried a wallet-size cardboard notebook with the bearer's name and address recorded on its face. This notebook was the patient's personal medical record. There were no hospital charts. The book listed previous hospital visits to Western and/or traditional clinics and gave short summaries of the patient's diagnoses and treatments.

In the dimly lit, concrete-lined corridors, patients sat and chatted about the usual things—a pain here, a good treatment one day, a bad treatment another day. They whispered about me, the "white-bearded foreigner." Some of the people sitting on the bench had been coming to this clinic for months or years or decades. These were our "regulars," the post-stroke patients, the arthritics, the chronic-pain patients, the perennial complainers. Every clinic in the world has its regular clients.

Occasionally, patients came from a distant city or province, self-referred, hoping for a dramatic cure of an incurable problem. When these travelers appeared, most of them farm workers dressed in peasant-style, padded black cotton outfits, the conversation turned to a discussion of the merits of city versus country life. Many patients also held strong views on the superiority of traditional medicine. Some even worried that the "treasure-house of traditional Chinese medicine"* might be lost to future generations as China modernized.

When a patient's number was called, he or she entered one of three treatment rooms. Zhang and I manned the first. Small children, relatives, and the occasional live chicken (purchased at the market on the way to the clinic) had to wait in the hall.

Our treatment room had a high ceiling, four six-foot fluorescent light fixtures, and plaster walls painted a glossy, light green. Twenty treatment tables, each five feet long, made the large space seem small. Zhang's desk was near the window. Next to it was a short, four-legged wooden stool. A series of metal shelves on the far wall supported aluminum boxes filled with reusable acupuncture needles. Beside the boxes were battery-driven electrical stimulators and herb sticks for moxibustion. The odor of burning moxa, very like marijuana's, permeated the room. Acupuncture charts covered every wall. One showed the points on the forearm; another dealt with points on the head and face; yet another displayed two hundred acupuncture points on the ear.

When a patient entered the treatment room, nineteen of the twenty tables were occupied. The patients on these tables had already told their stories, had had their needles inserted, and were now in the process of receiving a twenty- to forty-minute acupuncture treatment. The new patient sat on the stool alongside Zhang's desk and handed over his or her ticket and medical record book. Then Zhang proceeded to take a history. There was no privacy, no curtain, no soundproofing.

I was struck by the similarities between these patients and those I had cared for in the West. Each came to the clinic with an ordinary physical complaint and a unique collection of pre-

_____
* A descriptive phrase popularized by the late Chairman Mao.

conceptions, misconceptions, fears, and expectations. I kept a record of stories the patients told. By following the clinical course of fifty of our regular clients over a period of two months, I hoped to draw some preliminary conclusions about the use of acupuncture—not as an analgesic agent but as an age-old remedy for common illnesses.

The Stonemason

A sixty-two-year-old stonemason came in complaining of weakness in his right hand. His muscles and calluses attested to years of hard physical labor. He presented himself shyly to Dr. Zhang, his worker's cap clutched against his chest with both hands. He was a gentle man—a lovable grandpa who, except for bouts of high blood pressure, had never been sick a day in his life. The night before his arrival at the clinic, however, he had awakened with a tingling in his right hand. Within hours he could not move his hand. He had recovered some movement by now but still could not work his fingers normally.

Dr. Zhang attributed the condition to a minor stroke because of the patient's long-standing high blood pressure. Zhang told the man he would probably regain the use of his right hand.

Traditional medicine says that a stroke is a manifestation of excess "interior wind" and results from bodily imbalances in Yin and Yang. The old man seemed to think in this way. As he saw it, he had suffered a stroke in his brain—an excess of "interior wind" caused by an upset of the harmony in his outlook on life.

"Is it possible that I caused this stroke by thinking too much? I am a man of few thoughts. All my life I have been this way. It is just the way I am. Do you think, Dr. Zhang, that by thinking too much I damaged my brain? I thought a good deal over the

New Year's holiday. Thoughts about my children and grandchildren. Maybe this caused my stroke."

"No," said Zhang, "you must not blame yourself. We get old; these things happen. Let's see what we can do to correct the imbalances."

According to Chinese medicine, the common sequelae of stroke—such as paralysis, localized weakness (as in this case), numbness, and loss of speech—stem from the stagnation of Qi within meridians of the body. The stagnation results from the penetrating power of the "interior wind." The treatment for stroke and its sequelae seeks to clear the channels so as to facilitate the flow of Qi.

Two-inch needles were placed in the old man's hand, forearm, upper arm, and shoulder. The needles followed a line defined by the acupuncture channel associated with the "large intestine," and they also punctured a few points from the "triple burner" channel. Each time a needle was inserted and twisted, the old man would close his eyes and wait and nod when he had "obtained the Qi." He took fifteen needles in all. For thirty minutes the old stonemason sat there, staring at his lifeless right hand and mumbling to himself, "If only I had not strained these old brains of mine . . . if only I had not strained these brains . . ."

Over the next month the man received acupuncture treatments to his right arm three times a week. His grip improved about 50 percent. It remains unclear just how much the acupuncture influenced his recovery.

The Stroke Victim

A forty-eight-year-old man who had suffered right-sided paralysis from a recent stroke was more typical of the many stroke patients who came to the clinic. Although this man knew he had

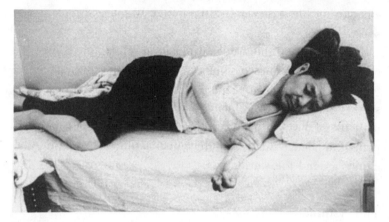

Treating a noncompliant stroke victim with acupuncture.

high blood pressure, he took few of the medications prescribed for him. He hated medicines, especially Western medicines, which he called poisons. He saw no point in taking medication unless he felt sick. Noncompliant hypertensive patients in the West echo the same sentiment. He smoked like a chimney, loved salt and spicy foods, admitted having a stressful job, but made no effort to seek other employment. Though he had had a stroke three years earlier, he recovered, and so didn't worry about the future until the second stroke hit.

The recent stroke temporarily cost him the use of his right arm and leg. He was unable to speak for days. Following his stroke, he began acupuncture treatment. Over the next few weeks, he made a remarkable recovery and once again attributed his improvement to the efficacy of the needles placed in his right foot, leg, hand, arm, and shoulder. It never occurred to this man that he might have recovered just as well without the acupuncture or that he might not have recovered even with the acupuncture. He refused to quit smoking, would not change his life-style, and still viewed Western drugs as poisons.

Stroke is one of the two leading causes of death in China (the other is cancer). Massive popular campaigns have been launched to control hypertension among China's vast population. This stroke victim was a problematical patient, not unlike difficult patients in Western medical clinics. Attempts to persuade this patient to change his ways failed, just as they often do in other clinics around the world.

The Asthmatic

A twenty-year-old woman with severe asthma was brought in by her mother. She had suffered from asthma her whole life. Recently, she had experienced asthmatic crises and worsening symptoms. I listened to her lungs with my stethoscope and heard the familiar wheezing of asthma. Dr. Zhang decided to treat this patient with a relatively new form of acupuncture.

The nervous young woman lay down on her back on one of the treatment tables. She unbuttoned her blouse and lowered her brassiere to expose her breastbone. Dr. Zhang cleansed the area around the breastbone with cotton dipped in alcohol. Then he asked for a scalpel. This surprised me; I had expected him to ask for a needle. Zhang told her to lie still, then took the blade and made a one-inch incision along her sternum. She winced. He took a pair of surgical clamps (hemostats) and used them to scrape the exposed surface of the bone. This must have been an excruciatingly painful procedure for the patient. Tears welled up in her eyes. After the scraping, Zhang applied a gauze bandage to the wound and instructed the woman to come back in a week for another treatment.

Before she got up, I listened to her lungs. I could detect no change from her pretreatment condition.

After the woman left, I asked Dr. Zhang why he hadn't used a topical anesthetic before making the incision in her chest.

"If I had used an anesthetic," he answered, "then the treatment would not have worked. If you ask me for proof, I have only my own experience and the experience of other acupuncturists."

I told him that the procedure seemed barbaric and that I would never be able to perform it on my own patients.

"But this is one of our most effective treatments," he said. "We can cure 70 to 80 percent of all asthmatic children using this method."

There was no way to verify this claim.

The twenty-year-old woman did not return for treatment for several weeks. Zhang assumed this meant her condition had responded to therapy. I took it to mean that she had been scared to death and would very likely not come back if her symptoms were severe enough to warrant the same treatment. When she finally returned, she was wheeze free. This time Zhang used acupuncture, not bone scraping, to try and strengthen her system and thereby prevent another asthma attack.

Zhang was not a cruel man. He did not enjoy the bone-scraping procedure. He used it only when he thought it would benefit his patient. He believed that it worked.

The Elderly Woman

The seventy-three-year-old Chinese woman was short and small, her face long and wrinkled. She wore black padded trousers, a black silk-lined jacket, and a preliberation hat made of crushed velvet and fine silk embroidery decorated with an opal pin. Tiny gold loop earrings hung from her ears in an age when few women dared wear jewelry in public. She walked into the clinic, went directly to the corner table, and began to disrobe.

Zhang leaned over and whispered to me, "This lady has been coming once or twice a week since the clinic opened in 1957!"

When I asked what was troubling her, she let forth a diatribe: "Did you say what's the matter? Look at my face! Do you see how horrible and old my face is? I am so old that my sons have already lost their teeth! I'm miserable! Miserable! It's useless to live any more. The Cultural Revolution did this to me! It ruined me, my family, everyone. And my stomach hurts. It hurts from early morning until I go to sleep at night. It will hurt until I die! Maybe it will hurt after I die! Here, feel here"—she placed my hand atop her belly—"here, doctor. Do your foreign fingers feel that tumor in there? That tumor is killing me!"

I couldn't feel any sign of a tumor. She continued.

"My legs hurt. And when it's windy, my body is influenced by the wind and sometimes my shoulders catch fire, and I can't move them! But my legs are the worst! The left one is more trouble than the right. Where are the needles? Why don't you needle me? I've been here for half a day talking to you, and nobody has taken up a single needle! I'm freezing here without my silk jacket! Do you know I've been coming here for twenty years? Needle me now!"

It was difficult to keep from laughing. Was I truly in the Beijing Institute of Traditional Chinese Medicine or was I in some Jewish Federation hospital in New York City? This woman reminded me of every complaining elderly Jewish lady I had ever cared for. She was a rice-fed yenta. Every part of her body was in pain, and she wanted or needed everyone to know this. I felt affection for this woman. I just wondered whether she would end her recital of afflictions in typical Jewish fashion: "So tell me, Sonny, are you married? I've got dis granddaughter vet would make sech a beautiful vife! . . ."

The Balding Lady

A twenty-six-year-old woman came in complaining of hair loss. She had heard that acupuncture cured baldness. I was interested in this patient's progress because if acupuncture could cure baldness, then there would surely be a minor cosmetological revolution in the West.

She said that baldness ran in her family. This was one strike against her. Since her teens, she had noticed that her hair was thinning evenly over her scalp. Strike two. She admitted that her hair was no thicker than her mother's, yet she insisted that her older sister had a "very thick head of hair." Strike three.

From a Western scientific standpoint, this sounded like a case of hereditary baldness. But the patient believed that her condition was due to the stressful work she had done since age seventeen and to her "personal struggle during the Cultural Revolution." She also speculated that her baldness might be related to a childhood case of rheumatic heart disease, to chronic "neurasthenia," or to other bodily imbalances.

Dr. Zhang cited a combination of family disposition and physical and psychological factors as possible causes for the baldness. He mentioned that acupuncture had been successful in treating baldness in *some* cases but that these had usually involved sudden hair loss. The condition of sudden hair loss is well recognized in the West, where it is called alopecia areata. In 80 to 90 percent of the cases, the patient's hair regrows spontaneously, without any treatment.

Dr. Zhang treated the woman with acupuncture, but he didn't build her hopes up. He used a special acupuncture device called a plum blossom needle—a small hammer with seven needles attached to its blunt claw. Zhang tapped the plum blossom lightly on her scalp, drawing a small amount of blood. This procedure normally takes up to an hour and involves the patient's entire scalp. It looked painful.

Unfortunately for her, but as expected, the treatment did not work for this patient. Her thinning hair and her beliefs remained unchanged.

The Retarded Child

I cannot forget a beautiful seven-year-old retarded girl with cerebral palsy who visited us for treatment. Her grandmother had carried her to the clinic every other day for five years. The little girl couldn't walk on her own. When she spoke, her words were garbled. In spite of her handicaps, she had a wonderful disposition. She laughed easily. Although she was unable to carry a tune or pronounce words clearly, she enjoyed singing children's songs and nursery rhymes. She struggled to control her voice, face, arms, and legs. Her smile after the completion of a song was a special gift to all of us in the clinic.

One day, as she was carried into the clinic, she said, *in English*, "Good morning, Dr. Ai. How are you today?" Her words were like an SOS—a tragic message from a beautiful soul imprisoned within an unresponsive shell of a body. She had learned her English sentence perfectly. Her grandmother ex-

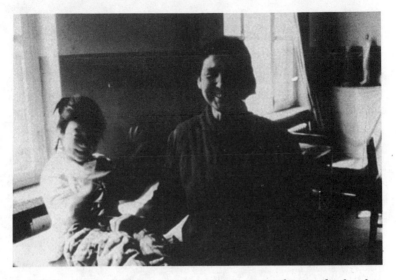

A child receives daily acupuncture treatments for cerebral palsy. Too much faith in acupuncture?

plained that the child's mother taught English at the Beijing Foreign Language Institute and that the child had memorized this sentence to surprise me. I assured the grandmother that I was both surprised and touched and asked her to thank the child's mother.

The girl had long since grown used to being needled every other day of her life. She barely flinched as the needles punctured her arms, legs, and face. During treatments, her grandmother stood by the bedside and held her hand. Two palms gripped one another and squeezed tightly as each needle pierced the little girl's skin. The grandmother was convinced that acupuncture had improved the girl's walking and talking.

Zhang cared a great deal about the little girl. He played and sang songs with her before and after each treatment. They were old friends. One day Zhang took the grandmother aside and said, "Comrade, I do not think acupuncture will undo all the problems of this child's neurological condition. She was born with them, and they will continue to make for a hard life." The grandmother listened politely. But she believed absolutely in the power of acupuncture. In her mind acupuncture had made the child more "normal" as she grew older. The possibility that her grandchild might have improved to a similar extent *without* acupuncture was not one she could envision, let alone accept.

The Commune Member

An unfortunate patient came to Beijing from Sichuan Province, two thousand miles away. Seven months earlier this commune member had begun losing strength in his arms. Subsequently, he lost strength in all his limbs, and his muscles wasted away with no apparent cause.

He had been seen initially by his local district doctors, who referred him to the provincial hospital for further evaluation. After tests the doctors had diagnosed a severe, degenerative neurological condition known as amyotrophic lateral sclerosis. They had said that the cause of this illness was unknown and that there was no effective treatment. They had advised the patient to return home with his family.

This man showed all the classic signs and symptoms—the muscle wasting, the twitching, and so forth—of amyotrophic lateral sclerosis (ALS), which in the West is also known as Lou Gehrig's disease. There exists no satisfactory (Western) therapy for ALS. The life expectancy of ALS sufferers is generally in the range of two to three years. The doctors in Sichuan Province had thus been accurate in their assessment of the patient's condition.

In search of some form of treatment, the patient's sons had carried him onto a train bound for Beijing to visit the famous

Beijing Capital Hospital, one of the finest Western-style hospitals in China (formerly called the Peking Union Medical College, founded by the Rockefeller Foundation). The doctors at the Beijing Capital Hospital agreed with the assessment of their medical colleagues in Sichuan. This was a case of ALS, and they knew of no therapy to reverse the condition. At this, the sons brought their father to Beijing's most renowned acupuncture clinic hoping that acupuncture would bring about a miraculous cure.

Zhang asked the sons to describe their father's illness from its onset. The elder son, wearing army greens, obviously on leave from active duty, sat on the familiar wooden stool and recounted the events. First he had noticed a peculiar emotional instability in his father; there were episodes of inappropriate laughter and inappropriate tears. Then the father began dropping things. The shovel slipped from his grasp; the plow overturned and was for the first time too heavy for him. When he lost control of his bladder function, he suffered tremendous humiliation and became withdrawn. It was then that his sons had carried him to the Sichuan hospital for an evaluation. While in the hospital, he lost the ability to pronounce words clearly. "This," said the elder son, "was the blow that crushed his spirit. This gave us the belief that we must try everything for him—even a trip to Beijing if there was a treatment for him there."

Zhang took hold of the man's left wrist and lifted it onto the desk to take his pulse. Then he examined the right wrist.

"Comrade, stick out your tongue." The commune worker could not obey the instruction, so Zhang gently separated the man's teeth and looked at his tongue. The elder son then lifted the patient onto the treatment table. His father lay on his side in a fetal position, his legs close to his chest. Zhang went to the back of the room and selected his needles. He placed more than twenty in the man's back, along his spine following the course of the bladder meridian. The patient's sensation was intact, and he could tell Zhang when he had "obtained the Qi" by nodding his head or uttering a guttural sound.

With needles in place, the man rested comfortably on the treatment table. Zhang approached the man's two sons and quietly asked how they paid for their medical expenses.

There are two types of medical insurance in China. One system covers factory workers and employees of state-run firms (banks, universities, shops). It is called the Labor Medical Insurance System and provides complete medical service to its recipients at no charge. It covers approximately 20 percent of China's population, primarily those living in urban areas. The unemployed receive no coverage.

The ALS patient belonged to the second insurance program, the Cooperative Medical Service. Eligible for this plan are the nearly 800 million Chinese who work on communes. Individual communes fund the Cooperative Medical Service through voluntary monthly payments by individual commune members. Reimbursement rates vary from 40 to 100 percent. A recent survey shows that only 40 to 45 percent of the rural population has *any* medical insurance at all.* The remaining 400 million Chinese have opted to use their health insurance money in other ways, chiefly as investment capital for their agricultural projects.

Noninsured Chinese can now turn to newly established private medical clinics for their health care needs. These local, for-profit, private practices are run by retired doctors or on the side by doctors working in state-run centers. These clinics have

* William Hsiao, "The Transformation of Health Care in China," *New England Journal of Medicine* 310 (1984): 932–36.

no ceilings on their earnings.* Whether this capitalistic innovation will flourish in China, no one can say.

In this instance, the ALS patient's commune reimbursed him for 50 percent of all required medical expenses. He had been reimbursed for 50 percent of his medical expenses from Sichuan hospitals, but he would receive no reimbursement for his medical expenses in Beijing. He was, after all, self-referred to Beijing.

The sons admitted that they had exhausted their family's savings in order to make the trip to Beijing and pay for their father's medical expenses. Zhang was very disturbed by this. He told the sons quite bluntly that he did not believe acupuncture could cure their father. He recommended they not waste more time or money in Beijing. It would be better for them to return home with their father so that he could die in peace and with dignity.

"Acupuncture, like all of man's medicine," said Zhang, "is not without its limitations. At times like this, we must remind ourselves of this." The sons accepted Zhang's advice and left Beijing that evening with their father.

Massage

Chinese therapeutic massage works on the same principles and uses the same anatomical points as acupuncture. The first person to give me a Chinese massage was totally blind. I met him during the summer of 1977 when I lived in Taiwan. Each night this blind man walked the neighborhood playing an eerie, high-pitched flute. Everyone recognized the sound. If you lived in that

---

* Christopher Wren, "China Turns to Private Practice to Heal System," *New York Times*, November 29, 1984.

small neighborhood of Taipei and needed a massage, you called out to the street when you heard the music. The blind old man would come into your home and, for $1.50, perform his magic.

The man's name was Zhu. He had been blind since birth from a congenital defect and was in his sixties when I met him. It is not uncommon for blind people in China to be trained in massage. This is a highly respected livelihood, and some of the finest massage masters throughout Chinese medical history have been blind.

My Taipei apartment, three floors above an old dim sum restaurant, was a one-bedroom sweatbox furnished with a plasterboard desk, two rattan chairs, and a three-inch-thick straw mattress. In the kitchen a rusted propane tank was connected to a makeshift cast-iron stove. The stove was for wok cooking and had three concentric circles of gas jets capable of bringing water to a boil within seconds. I used the flamethrower to make tea whenever Zhu arrived. He was, after all, a guest in my house.

After steeping a pot of tea, I followed Zhu's instructions and lay facedown, naked on my straw mattress. At the height of the summer typhoon season, whenever it wasn't raining, it was hot and humid. Zhu sat in the rattan chair, fanning himself and sipping tea, his gray eyeballs rolled back in his head. His cup finished, he sat silently for five or ten minutes while I lay motionless on the mat. He came down from the chair and positioned himself on his knees alongside me. Then his palms and fingertips scanned my body from head to toe, barely touching me. His hands were like electronic sensors. What he was trying to detect I could not imagine.

While barely making contact, he studied my neck and shoulders, back, buttocks, legs, and feet. After scanning two or three times, he began to push and pull and manipulate. Flesh, ligaments, and bones were putty in his hands. My muscles stretched and vertebrae cracked, and yet I felt no discomfort.

Suddenly, Zhu found what he was after: a tender point, a "trigger point"—one that, if pressed with just the right force, sent a deep ache radiating to my extremities.

" 'Spleen,' " he would mutter in Taiwanese while manipulating the trigger point between his thumb and forefinger. " 'Kidney,' " he'd say about the next point. "Another 'kidney' point," he'd go on. Each trigger point coincided with a particular acupuncture point along a specific meridian. Zhu was scanning my body by running his fingers along the tracks of the major acupuncture meridians. His diagnostic objective was to detect the trigger points that would best define the organ system primarily responsible for the bodily imbalance. His skill was in knowing which points were key.

Zhu selected a point on the left side of my neck and one on the left side of my lower back. I heard him take in a deep breath, and as he exhaled he began to apply pressure to these two points, using nothing but his fingertips. Then came a bizarre sensation of pressure and fullness and heat throughout my body. By the time Zhu withdrew his fingertips and began to use his palms to knead these points, I was already deeply relaxed. To be relaxed and at the same time aware of every nerve and muscle in your body is an unusual experience. To linger in this state for thirty or forty minutes was well worth $1.50. When Zhu was done, he drank a second cup of tea and departed.

At the Beijing Institute of Traditional Chinese Medicine three years later, I learned the theoretical principles behind Zhu's style of massage. The trigger points he searched for were perceived as temporary and reversible blockages of Qi along acupuncture meridians. The pushing and pulling of muscles, tendons, and bones was performed to reestablish or redirect the flow of Qi and re-create bodily harmony. By massaging and applying pressure to select points, the masseur could produce an improved physical state: it was acupuncture without the needles. That, at least, was the theory.

Dr. Sun Shu ran the massage clinic at the Dong Zhi Men Hospital. He was a stocky, cheerful man with huge hands and forearms the size of my legs. After graduating from the Beijing Traditional Medical College, Sun had specialized in therapeutic massage.

The first morning of class Dr. Sun came to my room at the institute carrying a fist-size beanbag filled with rice.

"Good morning, Dr. Ai," said Sun, punctuating his sentences by blowing air through his nose. He reminded me of a football coach.

"Good morning, Dr. Sun. Thank you for coming."

"Not at all. As you know, I have been asked to teach you something about massage these next few months."

"Yes. I've been looking forward to studying with you."

"I think we should begin by discussing the correct motion of the hands. You must learn to apply focused and sustained pressure to any part of the body using the fleshy portion of your palms or your fingertips. Here, watch."

Sun demonstrated on the rice beanbag. His wrist rotated from left to right while the base of his palm pushed against the bag. A few grains were crushed into white powder, which sifted through the porous cheesecloth.

"Here, you try it. Practice for three or four hours a day. When you can crush the entire bag to dust, then you will have gained the necessary strength and skill."

How absurd I felt sitting in my room in Beijing trying to crush rice into dust with my palms. My hands, wrists, and arms throbbed after only twenty minutes. That first week I produced no dust. Sun, by contrast, had made it look easy.

Daily classes consisted of rice crushing and my being massaged by Dr. Sun for two or three hours. No matter how much I ached from my rice workouts or running or Tai Ji Quan, Sun's magical hands brought relief and relaxation. For the first week he concentrated on my head, reviewing key acupuncture points and showing me where and how to apply pressure with my fingers. The next week he massaged my neck and back for several hours a day. Again he gave a detailed review of important points. This was my first lesson in finding trigger points.

Sun demonstrated that these points felt different from the surrounding soft tissues. They were circumscribed areas, firm nodules, or bands of muscles in spasm. When it came to trigger points, Sun's hands were forever on a seek-and-destroy mission. Having located a point, Sun applied staggering pressure to it with his fingertip or palm. This "acupressure" (identical to shiatsu) resulted in distant sensations of fullness exactly like those that acupuncture needling induced. This was the *de qi* phenomenon as manifest in massage. After applying point pressure for seconds or minutes, Sun would push and pull the surrounding muscles and skin using age-old hand and finger motions. This specialized pulling and rubbing of flesh is unique to massage therapy.

After each of Sun's massages I entered a state of relaxation and heightened awareness identical to the one I had experienced with the blind masseur in Taipei. Chinese massage impressed me as a valuable skill that, unlike most of traditional Chinese medicine, produced immediate and gratifying results.

As for the relation between massage and Qi, Sun maintained that Qi was the foundation of massage theory and practice. The competent masseur could feel the Qi in the trigger points and thereby know where and how to apply the correct massage technique.

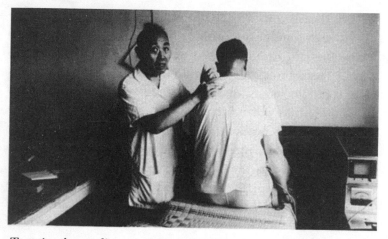

Treating heart disease with acupressure massage.

Treating Chef Hao in the massage clinic.

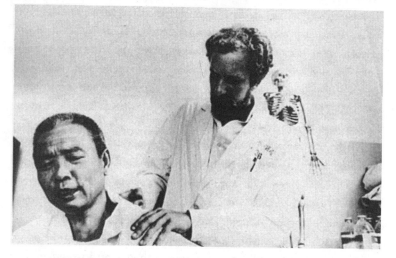

"That describes the competent masseur. The masters of massage," said Sun, "do not merely sense and redirect the flow of Qi; they transmit it from their own body into their patient's body by way of the appropriate meridian."

I began my work in the clinic after four weeks of rice crushing and classes during which Sun and I massaged one another. I helped treat more than one hundred patients over two months. Their complaints included headache, backache, sciatica, bone spurs, and slipped discs.

Every patient who entered that clinic felt dramatically relieved after thirty to sixty minutes of massage. There were no exceptions. The relief was typically short-lived, however, lasting hours to days, and the patients returned for further therapy.

Only controlled studies could prove whether Chinese massage altered the natural course of illness. Massage, like acupuncture, remains untested. It was unmistakably clear, however, that massage, when applied appropriately, made every patient markedly more comfortable and more relaxed, within minutes and without drugs. There is no reason why Western practitioners cannot learn and implement this skill. High technology and human touching are not mutually exclusive.

Acupuncture—An Effective Treatment for Which Diseases?

Beijing's clinic patients had the same illnesses, the same fears, the same hopes as patients in the West. What was different about the Beijing clinic was the age-old use of needles to treat those illnesses, fears, and hopes. Did the needles really make a difference?

Before its incarnation as a surgical analgesic, acupuncture had been used for more than two thousand years to treat nearly every disease known to man. *An Outline of Chinese Acupuncture,* a current reference text published by the Beijing Institute of Traditional Chinese Medicine, states that acupuncture is useful for the following disorders:

MEDICAL DISORDERS

cold/flu
bronchitis
asthma
heatstroke
peptic ulcers
gastric prolapse
hiccups
infectious hepatitis
acute diarrhea/dysentery
abdominal pain
palpitations
coronary heart disease
shock
rheumatic heart disease
Ménière's syndrome
vertigo/dizziness
hypertension
cerebrovascular accident
   (thrombosis, embolism,
   hemorrhage, retardation)

urinary-tract infection
neurasthenia
schizophrenia
epilepsy
headaches
trigeminal neuralgia
facial paralysis
intercostal neuralgia
numbness
nephritis
arthritis
malaria
posttraumatic paraplegia
sciatica
diabetes
local nerve damage
pneumonia
impotence/spermatorrhea
brachial plexus damage

SURGICAL DISORDERS

appendicitis
biliary-tract disease
ruptured ulcer
mastitis
tetanus
erysipelas
furuncle
lymphangitis
hyperthyroid/goiter
tuberculosis
rectal prolapse
hemorrhoids

urticaria
neurodermatitis
stiff neck
back pain
shoulder pain
elbow pain
wrist pain
tenosynovitis
knee pain
ankle pain
heel pain
hair loss

OBSTETRICAL AND GYNECOLOGICAL DISORDERS

oligomenorrhea/amenorrhea
dysmenorrhea
menorrhagia
leukorrhea
uterine prolapse

morning sickness
fetal maldistribution
prolonged labor
lactation deficiency
pelvic inflammatory disease

PEDIATRIC DISORDERS

whooping cough
failure to thrive
seizures

mumps
polio/paralysis

SENSE ORGAN DISORDERS

conjunctivitis
nearsightedness
glaucoma
optic atrophy
tonsillitis/pharyngitis

sinusitis
deafness
mutism
toothache
rhinitis, tinnitus

My direct experience was limited to the patients I helped treat in the acupuncture clinic of the Dong Zhi Men Hospital over three months. In that clinic, patients complained primarily of neurological, psychiatric, or musculoskeletal problems. The chief complaints of sixty consecutive patients are summarized below:

NEUROLOGICAL COMPLAINTS	(47%)	PAIN-RELATED	(21%)
stroke	18	knee pain	4
numbness	10	headache	3

NEUROLOGICAL COMPLAINTS *(cont.)*	(47%)	PAIN-RELATED *(cont.)*	(21%)
retardation	5	backache	2
facial paralysis	3	sciatica	2
deafness	3	abdominal pain	2
dizziness	2	shoulder pain	2
trigeminal neuralgia	1	arthritis	1
nearsightedness	1	wrist pain	1
epilepsy	1	ankle pain	1
enuresis	1	heel pain	1
paraplegia	1	neck pain	1
nerve damage trauma	1	elbow pain	1

PSYCHIATRIC COMPLAINTS	(23%)	MISCELLANEOUS	(9%)
neurasthenia	17	hair loss	3
hysteria	2	allergy	2
schizophrenia	2	gastric ulcer	2
emotional disturbance	2	conjunctivitis	1
		asthma	1

By following these patients over time (anywhere from one week to twelve weeks), I hoped to measure acupuncture's efficacy in treating common medical problems. Did acupuncture alter what Western medicine calls the natural course of illness?

The "natural course of illness" refers to the expected outcome in a given patient of a given, untreated illness. For instance, if a patient suffers a hypertensive stroke that leaves him paralyzed, what are the chances of his regaining muscular or sensory function if nothing is done? The answer to this question requires the tracing of data from hundreds or thousands of untreated stroke victims over time. The "natural course" defines a set of probabilities deduced from the observation of many patients with the same illness. Without some biostatistical understanding of an illness's natural course, it is impossible to know whether a given therapeutic intervention is better or worse than no intervention at all.

Traditional Chinese medicine evolved without biostatistics and without the "natural course of illness" concept. This partly explains the confusion and mistrust between doctors of Western and Chinese medicine. For example, if most stroke patients receive acupuncture treatment following their strokes, and if most of them get better over time, does this necessarily mean that acupuncture is effective in treating stroke patients? No. Does it mean that acupuncture is ineffective? No. One cannot make a judgment without designing an appropriate study that compares the outcomes of stroke treatments using acupuncture therapy with those of treatments not using it. Such a study must also guarantee that belief systems and personal biases do not interfere with the results. This is complicated work, requiring large numbers of patients, meticulous study design, and sophisticated mathematics.

Most of the patients I followed in the acupuncture clinic improved, but they did so gradually, over a period of months. This exploded my hope that acupuncture would prove to be as impressive as a treatment for common illness as it was for surgical pain. During each clinic session, I vainly awaited the miraculous response—the patient who would enter with incapacitating pain or wheezing and who after a single treatment by Dr. Zhang would leave the clinic with the words "Thank you, Doctor. All of my symptoms are gone now." In the same way that earlier twentieth-century physicians put their faith in the new wonder drugs like sulfa (magic bullets, as they were called), I wanted to put my faith in needles that I hoped would cure a multitude of illnesses. Acupuncture massage produced immediate results that did not last. Acupuncture produced modest results only over a long course of treatment.

Dr. Zhang thought my expectations for acupuncture were inappropriate and unrealistic. "Acupuncture," he said, "promotes the body's ability to augment recovery over a period of time. Remember that it takes time to reach the *root* of an illness, and only rarely can this occur in the dramatic fashion you hoped to see."

With acupuncture therapy and time, patients' neurological problems resolved, their musculoskeletal pains diminished, and their anxiety levels decreased. But because there were no untreated patients to compare them with—no "control groups"—it was impossible to know whether acupuncture was directly responsible for these clinical improvements. Acupuncture may in fact be superior to standard Western therapy in a variety of common illnesses, but without appropriate clinical studies no Western scientist will be convinced.

Acupuncture—Unanswered Questions, Unproven Assertions

There is sufficient scientific evidence to confirm that acupuncture can predictably and reproducibly alter pain perception in animals and in humans, but a physiological explanation for this phenomenon remains incomplete. A look at a select group of Chinese acupuncture patients may bring us closer to a solution. Every acupuncture clinic in Beijing and Shanghai reported patients who were "addicted" to acupuncture needling. Experienced acupuncturists recognized them easily. These patients complained vaguely of headaches, abdominal pain, or anxiety and insisted on extensive full-body acupuncture. They visited the clinics several times a week, asking for more needles, longer needles, and more time on the treatment table. Without acupuncture, these men and women became agitated, nervous, and difficult to manage. They experienced a physical hell not unlike that associated with narcotic withdrawal. If acupuncture induces the production and/or secretion of morphine-like substances within the brain, it is conceivable that these patients were addicted to these substances. They were apparently exquisitely sensitive to the process of acupuncture. A more detailed study of these individuals may show the way to an improved biochemical explanation for acupuncture analgesia.

It is worth speculating about the similarity between acupuncture "addiction" and the increasingly common phenomenon of "addiction to exercise." Many exercise enthusiasts, particularly long-distance runners, feel unwell if they miss their regular exercise. Like the acupuncture "addict," these highly trained athletes experience generalized malaise, headache, insomnia, and the like if they stop exercising. The common ground here may be the effects of acupuncture and exercise on endorphins, the body's own opiates.

There is no Western scientific proof that acupuncture points or meridians exist as physical entities. Anatomical studies have failed to reveal discrete channels or neuromuscular points coinciding with the detailed maps used by acupuncturists. Once again, the Chinese claim to have discovered a select group of patients that may clarify this situation. According to published reports from the Beijing Institute of Traditional Chinese Medicine, approximately one in a thousand acupuncture patients will experience a unique series of sensations while undergoing acupuncture. These patients experience a "propagation of sensation along acupuncture channels." Documentary films made by the institute show a series of three patients who, once needled, report a sensation of "fullness" or "electrical shock" propagating at a very slow speed along specific tracts covering their body. According to Chinese physiologists, these sensations are accompanied by neuromuscular changes that can be tracked by nerve conduction studies.

The paths of these neuromuscular changes allegedly coincide with the acupuncture meridians that the first Chinese physicians defined thousands of years ago. Traditional Chinese medical authorities insist that acupuncture channels exist as physical entities. They use the observation of "propagation along acupuncture channels" as proof of this claim.

Another problem concerns the question of how to induce acupuncture stimulation. There is no consensus on the best way to accomplish this. The ancients used needles of gold or stone. Today the Chinese are experimenting with numerous stimulation techniques, including a variety of metal and synthetic needles, low-voltage electricity, pressure, laser beams, sonar rays, and injections of water or steroids. At present there is no clinical confirmation that any one method is superior to another.

The biggest problem lies in convincing Western-style clinicians—the rank-and-file medical and surgical doctors practicing in the United States, in Europe, and in *China*—that acupuncture does more than alter pain thresholds, that it does more than provide analgesia for a select group of Chinese patients, and that it can be used effectively, reliably, and safely on patients. To convince doctors of Western medicine of acupuncture's efficacy will take more than testimonials by patients or films of successful operations. It will require well-designed clinical studies probably best done first in China under the supervision of Western research experts. If acupuncture really works, then it should work better than no treatment at all, better than sham (or incorrectly applied) acupuncture, better than a placebo. Without stud-

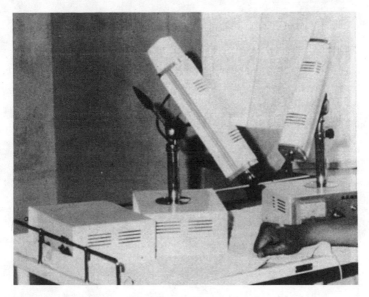

Laser acupuncture. The three-thousand-year-old controversy about how best to stimulate acupuncture points continues.

ies to confirm acupuncture's clinical efficacy, reliability, and safety, there will be no referrals between conventional Western doctors and acupuncturists. There will be no mutual understanding and no integration. The current limbo will continue.

In the Clinic:
Herbal Medicine

Down the green corridor from the acupuncture clinic in the Dong Zhi Men Hospital lies a warehouse of strange-smelling substances. Six hundred wooden drawers, each the size of a breadbox, line the gigantic room from floor to ceiling. Subdivided and labeled, the drawers hold thousands of plant, animal, and mineral substances. These are the medicines that traditional doctors prescribe.

Twenty pharmacists in white lab coats and caps work in the middle of this room at a long table. They scurry from drawer to drawer, measuring the weights of each medication on hand scales, before placing them on large trays. At the workbench, they mix and pour the medications onto brown squares of wrapping paper. Each resulting bundle contains a precise amount of a dozen or so herbs, roots, powders, and animal remains. It has

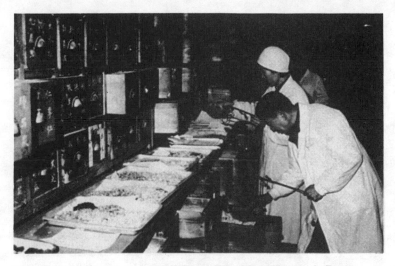

The herbal pharmacy of the Dong Zhi Men Hospital, Beijing.

been so in the Chinese pharmacy, and no different, for roughly two thousand years.

At the entrance to the pharmacy opposite the main reception counter, the patients wait in line to drop off their prescriptions and receive voucher coupons that they will use when they pick up and pay for their medications. Chinese herbal pharmacists must decipher the ancient, stylized calligraphy of traditional prescription writing. Their task corresponds to that faced by pharmacists who must decipher the illegible scribble of American doctors.

Herbal medicines (*cao yao*—literally, "medicine from plants") constitute the principal method of traditional medical intervention, far outweighing acupuncture or massage. Older Chinese in urban centers and the 800 million people in the countryside prefer traditional herbal medicines to Western drugs. Western

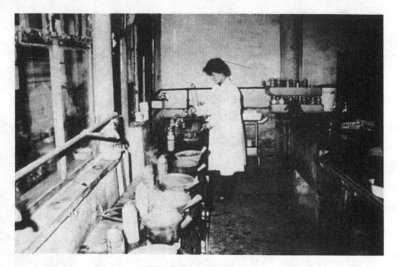

Preparing herbal prescriptions to be carried in Thermoses to hospitalized patients on the medical wards.

medicines, the feeling seems to be, are fast-acting, powerful remedies that have dangerous side effects. Herbal preparations, by contrast, are more natural, far less dangerous, slower and gentler in action, but equally or more effective.

China's vast pharmacopoeia contains more than two thousand substances of plant, animal, or mineral origin. Most are herbs, but there are also deer antlers, snake gall bladders, shark fins, and numerous other curious substances. Each medication is graded on the basis of where it was harvested, how it was processed, and so on. Some are unbelievably expensive. For example, the highest-grade ginseng root, graded in part on its resemblance to the human body, can cost hundreds of dollars an ounce.

An herbal prescription usually contains between six and twelve medicines. One prepares it by boiling the leaves or powder in water in a pot made from a special clay. The mixture must simmer at a specified heat for a specified time, before it is strained and drunk. The broth makes a hot herbal tea unpalatable to most Westerners. Outpatients have caldrons at home and can boil their own prescriptions. Inpatients rely on the pharmacy to weigh, boil, strain, and decant their daily herbal prescriptions, which the nursing staff carries to the hospital wards in small Thermoses.

Physicians of traditional Chinese medicine recognize herbal therapy as the most complex and demanding medical subspecialty. In order to prescribe herbal remedies effectively, one must first master Chinese medical theory as well as tongue and pulse diagnosis. The dependable recall of thousands of combinations of well-studied herbal preparations is the next prerequisite. Add these skills to twenty or thirty years of experience and you get a respected herbal doctor. The one I met was Dr. Weng.

Weng was a jocular, middle-aged man with a white crew cut, baggy pants, a long doctor's coat, and a very elegant quill-tipped pen. He was the director of the Dong Zhi Men Pharmacy and a scholar on the subject of Chinese medical-drug interaction. Weng was also a gourmet chef.

"Great food," he used to tell me, "must be prepared like great prescriptions, following ancient guidelines, using the finest ingredients, concocted with consummate skill."

Weng saw food as an extension of herbal medicine. "Everything we eat is a kind of medicine," he said. "Every substance has its own influence on excesses and deficiencies in our bodies. Certain foods are more influential than others, particularly when they themselves are excessively Yin or Yang by nature. For a given patient, certain foods would be unwise to eat, while others would offer a profoundly therapeutic effect."

My diet was the full-time responsibility of Comrade Hao, a

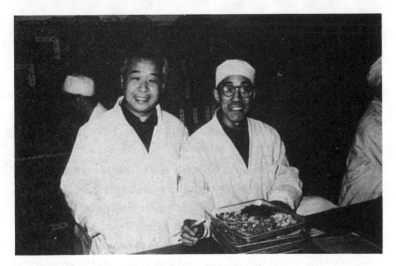

Dr. Weng (left), a specialist in herbal medicine.

chef at the institute. Hao had been assigned to cook for the foreign guests living in my small courtyard. Chef Hao and Dr. Weng were close friends, and they appreciated the nuances of banquet-style cooking, the colors, the aromas, the choice of spices, the ornate vegetable carvings, and the need for a balanced presentation and, above all, for a careful attention to the harmony of Yin and Yang within each meal.

Hao, a rotund fellow with a stubbly white beard, had a passion for fine food, good wine, and American cigarettes. His white apron was indelibly stained with garlic, soy sauce, ginger root, and tobacco ashes. He was a master chef, able to prepare dishes in any provincial style. Before his assignment at the institute, he had been a cooking instructor; the only thing Hao liked doing more than cooking was teaching others to cook.

My father and his father had been professional bakers and extraordinary chefs. Cooking was in my blood, and I had studied it most of my life, though I didn't think it had much to do with medicine.

Most of the meals we cooked together were simple, made from vegetables, bean curd, rice, noodles, and a small amount of chicken or fish. This diet was high in carbohydrate and low in saturated fat and cholesterol. Once or twice a week Hao and I dreamed up an "advanced class." At the Beijing Friendship Store (where only foreign guests are allowed to shop), I had access to fresh fish, duck, shrimp, crab, exotic spices, mushrooms, and fungus. In Hao's kitchen, just a few feet from my courtyard, these ingredients were chopped, steamed, sautéed, and sculpted into culinary extravaganzas. There was no point in my going to restaurants. I lived in one.

"Every dish," said Dr. Weng, "is subtly spiced and garnished with key ingredients. This is not so different from a medical prescription. It just so happens that certain foods in combination with key ingredients are tastier than others. [For example, ginger root, orange peel, star anise, and barley have medicinal powers.] The difficulty is in knowing which ingredients, herbs, and rare spices should be used in a given situation to improve bodily harmony. This requires study and experience."

Gourmet cooking and herbal medicine both originate in the Daoist philosophy of Yin and Yang. They are extreme applications of the hypothesis that we are what we eat. In traditional medical theory Qi, the life force, comes from only three sources —heredity, air, and food. It follows that in order to maintain health and a harmony of Qi, one must consume the correct foods and herbs.

The question remains, How applicable is this 2,500-year-old theory to the modern world? How effective are the potions? The herbal clinic where Dr. Weng and I saw patients was on the second floor of the hospital, just above the pharmacy. In a central waiting area more than one hundred patients sat on lacquered wooden benches beneath bigger-than-life photographs of Hua Guo-feng (then premier) and Mao Ze-dong. Two long hallways connected ten examining rooms to the central area. A nurse dressed in a long white coat, white blouse, and cotton cap called out numbers as patients were escorted into the examining rooms. These rooms were cubicles measuring six by eight feet and containing a single desk and two chairs, one for the patient and the other for the doctor. The walls were of cracked concrete and plaster, the fluorescent fixtures were sparse, and the heating was nonexistent. On gray winter mornings the clinic was a cold, dimly lit place.

More than one thousand patients came each day. Their chief complaints differed from those I had catalogued in the acupuncture and massage clinics. They tended to be common medical problems rather than neurological or musculoskeletal problems. For example, these patients complained of dizziness, headache, shortness of breath, impotence, diarrhea, weakness, and rash. The same complaints could be seen in any medical walk-in clinic in the West. Patients seemed to know which of the traditional medical subspecialties—acupuncture, massage, or herbal medicine—would be most appropriate as an initial therapy for a given condition.

Of the fifty patients I followed in this clinic over a two-month period, a twenty-seven-year-old man with ulcerative colitis was the most memorable. He was a 220-pound, chain-smoking weight lifter who habitually flexed his biceps and spat while he talked. His attitude was anxious and his speech pressured; although he had an imposing muscular frame, his "macho" veneer was thin. He was obviously scared. This fellow had suffered from ulcerative colitis since his late teens. Intermittent cramping pains, fever, and bloody diarrhea were the initial symptoms. A biopsy taken at a major Western-style teaching hospital in Beijing confirmed the diagnosis of ulcerative colitis. At age twenty, part of this man's colon had been removed because of a severe flare-up of his condition. He had been stable for the next seven years, but lately, for two to three weeks, he'd noted the return of his symptoms. On the day he visited our clinic, he complained of two weeks of pain, fever, and ten to fifteen bloody bowel movements per day. His former doctors at the Beijing Western hospital recommended immediate hospitalization and removal of the remainder of his colon. These recommendations had panicked the patient. "You must help me," he said to Dr. Weng, "I have cried a sea of tears, and will do anything to avoid the torture of another operation. Please help me. You are my only chance."

Weng listened patiently without comment. When the man was finished, Weng asked questions about the quality of the man's fevers and sweats and about his appetite, his mood, and his ability to see and think clearly. Then Weng studied the man's face as he kept his hands on his lap and stared at the floor. After a long silence, Weng tapped the table with his forefinger. Responding to cue, the young man thrust his wrist before Weng's hand. With the three fingers of his right hand, Weng touched the man's left wrist. He took the pulse there, then on the opposite wrist. Weng felt the pulse like a safecracker. He closed his eyes; he felt, heard, timed, and sensed twelve pulses in all. "Let me see your tongue," Weng said. The young man put his tongue forward as far as it would reach. Again, careful, silent study, for more than a minute.

The examination was over. Weng had come to a diagnosis: the man had a primary deficiency of Qi involving the "spleen." He took out his quill pen and wrote an ancient prescription. The names of the following nine medicines were written in beautiful calligraphy:

12 grams	peony root	*(Paeonia lactiflora Pull)*
9 grams	fan feng	*(Ledebouriella seseloides Wolff)*
9 grams	mandarin orange peel	*(Citrus reticulata Blanco)*
9 grams	pai shu	*(Atractylodes macrocephala Koidz)*
9 grams	pagoda tree	*(Sophora japonica)* L.
9 grams	burnet bloodwort	*(Sanguisorba officinalis)* L.
9 grams	Chinese palm (petiole fiber)	*(Trachycarpus fortunei H. Wendl.)*
9 grams	meadow rue	*(Thalictrum foliolosum DC.)*
9 grams	licorice	*(Glycyrrhiza uralensis Fisch)*

"Your condition has been studied for hundreds of generations. The prescription I have written you was recommended by the famous Dr. Li Shi-jen in the year 1578 and is still the most effective. You are to simmer it in a clay pot for forty minutes. Drink the herbal liquid three times a day. Here is enough for one week's time. Come back and see me then, because as your condition changes you will need another prescription for a different combination of herbs. You will be all right. Try and rest. Try and smoke less. Do not drink alcohol. You must seek out friends or family who can give you a sense of peace, and not nervousness. Do not understand?"

"Yes I do. I will try. I will do anything to avoid the surgeon's knife."

"Excuse me," I interrupted, "would you mind keeping a diary over the next week and writing down all of your symptoms including bowel movements every day?"

"Yes, I can do this," the young man answered.

In a Western medical facility, the evaluation and management of this patient would have been entirely different. He would have had blood tests and an extensive physical examination. It would have been necessary to determine the extent of the man's blood loss and rule out the possibility of a serious infection. He would probably have been hospitalized immediately and treated with antibiotics and other medications. His doctors would also have considered surgery, particularly since ulcerative-colitis patients who do *not* have their colons removed face a significant risk of developing colon cancer. Instead, he went home with a brown paper bag filled with dried leaves and roots and with instructions to relax.

In Western terms this patient had ulcerative colitis. In Chinese terms the patient's intestinal problems were a manifestation of a " 'spleen' deficiency"—for example, a primary deficiency of the digestive system. Not all patients labeled by Western doctors as having ulcerative colitis would be diagnosed by traditional Chinese medicine as having "primary deficiencies of the 'spleen.' " Some might have excesses or deficiencies of other organs that result in ulcerative colitis. The age-old prescription used in this instance would not be applicable to all ulcerative colitis patients. Moreover, the nine herbs prescribed initially would need to be changed in days or weeks, depending on the patient's response.

A week later the man reappeared in our clinic.

"How have you been?" asked Weng.

"You are the most powerful doctor there is. You have made me well. It is unbelievable to me and everyone in my family. Not even the doctors in the other hospital believe it."

"Tell me, what about the pain and bloody diarrhea?" asked Weng.

The man took out his diary. Within three days after he had started taking herbal medicines, the man's pain had subsided and the bloody diarrhea decreased from fifteen to three times per day. Over the next four days, the bleeding had stopped altogether, the pain vanished, and the frequency of bowel movements returned to normal. This was a remarkable and impressive recovery for someone suffering a severe flare-up of ulcerative colitis.

Weng again listened to the man's symptoms, repeated his tongue and pulse diagnosis, and wrote out an altogether different prescription, including several different herbal remedies. This prescription was meant to "tonify" the man's state of balance and prevent a flare-up of the ulcerative colitis. Once again, Weng advised the patient to change his life-style and be temperate in his activities.

What had happened to explain this patient's unusual recovery? Perhaps the herbs contained active ingredients that were directly responsible. Maybe the recovery was due to a placebo effect based on the man's belief that these herbs would help him. It is also possible that the doctor-patient relationship—the reassurance, the supportive tone—somehow changed this young man physically and that this, in turn, altered the natural course of his illness. The patient's change in life-style or mental attitude may have contributed as well. Or perhaps a combination of these explanations is correct. The trouble is we do not know, because we rarely ask these questions, rarely go to the trouble of designing appropriate tests to determine cause-and-effect relations.

Do not imagine that we have the answers to these questions as they pertain to all *Western* drugs either. We do not. The over-the-counter pill you take for your cold or dizziness often works, *if* it works, through mechanisms that are not understood. Hundreds of Western drugs work in unknown ways and may well require a combination of active ingredients, placebo effects, and doctor-patient or mind-body interactions in order to achieve a therapeutic effect. Western medical science is only beginning to investigate this complex and crucial aspect of the healing process.

My observations of patients in the herbal-medicine clinic paralleled the ones I made in the acupuncture and massage clinics. Chinese patients presented the same problems as medical patients in the West. They had the same symptoms of congestive heart failure, the same depression, dizziness and weakness, and the same problems of impotency, infertility, menstrual cramping, and excessive bleeding. The patients were the same, but the Chinese approach to diagnosis and therapy was very different. Chinese diagnoses described abnormal states of Yin and Yang, Qi, "blood," and organ imbalance. Laboratory tests were nonexistent. Prescriptions were unintelligible to me, and they were changed constantly on the basis of the patient's symptoms and tongue and pulse diagnosis. However, sick patients showed marked improvement over time. Some improvement, such as that of the man with ulcerative colitis, was dramatic. In other instances it was gradual. The dramatic responses are nothing more than anecdotal case reports. Without looking at large numbers of patients and comparing one kind of therapy with another under controlled conditions, it is impossible to know the overall effectiveness of herbal remedies.

Hundreds of clinical studies of the efficacy of herbal medicines in treating everything from heart disease to cancer have been undertaken in recent years. Most of these studies have been published exclusively in Chinese, and many have been fundamentally flawed by poor study design. Others have failed because of the high variability of herbs grown and processed in different parts of China. The studies have faced the additional problem of isolating the *active* ingredients within an herbal mixture containing hundreds of ingredients. The research continues without a consensus on the clinical efficacy of herbal medicine in the prevention or treatment of common medical problems.

Acupuncture, herbal medicine, and massage are considered nonconventional therapeutic techniques by doctors of Western medicine. These nonconventional therapies are nevertheless used by millions of Americans and Europeans and hundreds of millions of Chinese. Western-style physicians rarely refer patients to acupuncturists or herbalists and frequently refuse to share medical records with these nonconventional health care providers. The practice of nonconventional therapy continues, however, in an atmosphere of noncommunication between practitioners of Chinese and Western medicine.

My observations in the clinics of a Beijing hospital suggest that acupuncture, herbal medicine, and massage may be highly effective therapeutic tools. How reliable, reproducible, and effective they are and whether they work directly or indirectly is not known. Doctors of Western medicine and doctors of Chinese medicine share the responsibility of applying rigorous scientific methods to the study of these techniques. If traditional Chinese medical practices can be shown to be more effective than Western medical techniques in preventing or treating specific illnesses, then doctors of Western medicine must make themselves aware of this and refer their patients accordingly. By the same token, if Western doctors can prove to the satisfaction of their non-Western medical colleagues that certain traditional medical practices do not work, then these practices should be discontinued. For doctors of Western medicine and doctors of traditional Chinese medicine to avoid one another, because of the misconception that neither school of thought has anything to offer the other, is an act of ignorance and arrogance. In the end the patients suffer most from this narrow-mindedness.

Doctors of Western medicine and doctors of traditional Chinese medicine have much to learn by comparing practices and by testing one another. It is time for an exchange of medical information and positive criticism. Condescension and bias need to be unlearned and replaced with mutual cooperation and intensive investigation.

Third Encounter:
The Qi Gong
Masters

Qi Gong masters were considered state secrets in 1979. In that year Beijing's "democracy wall" was dismantled and numerous Chinese were imprisoned for sharing "state secrets" with foreigners. Some of my colleagues were eager to satisfy my curiosity about Qi Gong masters, and I feared that this might cause them political trouble.

One day a friend called. "Dr. Ai," he said, "please meet me in the alleyway alongside the medical institute at one o'clock sharp. It is very important."

"But, I have an acupuncture class at one," I said; "maybe we can arrange to meet at . . ." Before I could finish, he hung up.

When I met my friend in the deserted alley, he told me that a Qi Gong master visiting from a distant province had heard of my interest in Qi and was willing to meet me. I said I would welcome any such opportunity, and my friend waved his hand;

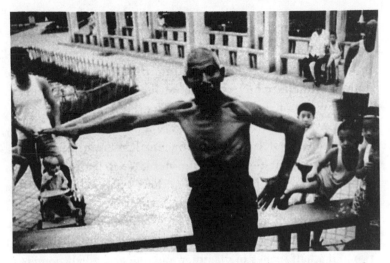

An anonymous Qi Gong master performing for a street crowd.

the Qi Gong master suddenly appeared at the end of the alley-way.

He stood before me, his eyes deep-set and dark, opened just a fraction of an inch wider than the eyes of an ordinary person. His forearms would have made Popeye jealous. At sixty, his skin was taut. His shaven head had multiple scars. Above and beyond his apparent physical strength, this man possessed an aura of confidence and calm defiance—Buddhist monk and man of steel combined. He looked as though he could meditate peacefully for hours after eating a box of nails. The Qi Gong master shook my hand and introduced himself. Then he said, "Please find a rock. Any rock."

I walked to the end of the alleyway and picked up a stone about four inches thick and twice as long. He studied the rock in his hand, then put it on a concrete doorstep. He looked at me with a mesmerizing glance, inhaled three times, and with his left fist dealt the stone one sharp blow. It broke neatly in half and rolled off the concrete doorstep.

A small crowd of neighborhood children had by then gathered to watch the Qi Gong master perform. He had not wished to be noticed. He told me to meet him at his cousin's that evening. "Bring plenty of rocks," he said. Then he left.

That evening proved to be one of the most memorable of my life. As soon as I had entered the small room of his cousin's modest apartment, the Qi Gong master began to perform. He was determined to convince me that Qi does exist and that all the stories I had heard about Qi Gong were true.

He started with his daily warm-up exercises, designed to help him gain control of his Qi. First he swallowed an iron ball, about two and a half inches in diameter and one and a half pounds in weight. Then he swallowed another. He invited me to feel for the two spheres in his stomach. I probed his belly and palpated two metallic lumps. He then brought up the balls against gravity, spitting them at my feet. Quite a warm-up. He told me that some Qi Gong masters practice this routine with as many as six iron balls. Those who specialize in this skill use their Qi to project the balls a distance of yards. The Qi Gong master then reached for one of my fist-size stones and cracked it against his head at his hairline.

I feared that this odd man would overdo the rock-smashing activities and break his skull open right in front of me. It was a ghastly vision. I told him I was more interested in the emission of Qi than in its application to the smashing of objects. What I really wanted, I told him, was to see a Qi Gong master move an inanimate object without touching it.

The Qi Gong master put the stones away and sat down to reflect. "I've never tried that before," he said. "I can fight off fifteen trained men at one time. I can use my Qi to repel them.

But I've never aimed my Qi at inanimate objects before. I'll try. What shall I move?"

I looked around the room and pointed to a Chinese lantern hanging from the ceiling. It was four feet tall and contained six sections of hand-cut glass held together by strips of hardwood. Six long red tassels hung from its base, and a candle flickered at its center.

The Qi Gong master suggested that the tassels would serve as his opponents. He would attempt to set his Qi in motion, direct it through his arm into his palm, then fire at the tassels from three feet away. He walked through his paces once in slow motion to show me where he expected to finish. From that point, three feet away from the lantern, I tried to make the tassels move by fanning them with my hands. By waving my hands wildly, I could barely influence the two tassels nearest me. The other four remained motionless.

The Qi Gong master was ready. He began his deep breathing and started straining and contorting his muscles by initiating a short series of martial arts steps similar in form to Tai Ji Quan. From the waist up, his shoulders, arms, and hands traced circles in the air. From the waist down, his body was anchored like a root in the earth. At the end of his gesturing, his left foot and right arm pointed directly at the lamp. The fingers of his right hand were relaxed, and his palm was perpendicular to the tassels. Then it happened. Though he was three feet away, the tassels moved—all six of them. Slowly, the lantern began to swing back and forth. I was speechless. Either I had been tricked or this was my first exposure to forces that Western science had not yet defined.

The Qi Gong master sat down, exhausted. He asked me whether I would like to see him smash a few more rocks. I told him to relax. It was one thing to train people to break rocks or

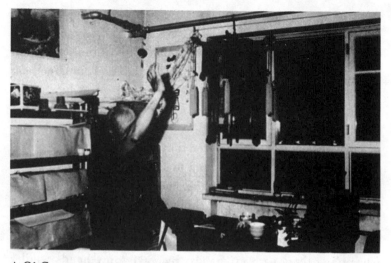

A Qi Gong master moves a lantern with external Qi. "Emitting Qi is like exhaling."

bear concrete slabs on their chests. But moving inanimate objects without touching them was another thing altogether. When a Qi Gong master smashed a rock, was he using his physical strength alone or his physical strength coupled with Qi? Could he really repel people with this Qi? Did acupuncturists truly send Qi through their needles? Did people who studied Qi Gong actually possess unique powers?

The Qi Gong master shared his thoughts. He believed absolutely in the existence of Qi, but he knew that some Qi-related claims of supernatural strength were false. Some Qi Gong feats were easy; others required a lifetime of dedication. He himself did not understand all of them. He told me about the Qi Gong stunts that were unrelated to Qi. For instance, certain Qi Gong practitioners balanced their bodies against pointed spears by depending on the angle of the spearhead to protect them from being pierced. No Qi Gong master, he said, could make his skin impenetrable to sharp objects. Lesser Qi Gong masters gave the illusion of breaking massive stones by selecting those that could be broken most easily. In these instances they relied on physical strength, calluses, and their knowledge of stress points. On the other hand, this was not true of the great Qi Gong masters, who used their Qi as well as their physical power to crack enormous blocks of stone.

A Qi Gong master could perform feats that relied heavily on Qi and only minimally on physical strength. The moving of an inanimate object was a good example. He said he could feel the Qi flowing in his body, but he did not pretend to understand its power: "It is inside of me. It is a part of me, like an arm or a breath. Can you explain what it is like to exhale? Emitting Qi is like exhaling for me. Can anyone fully understand a breath?"

While continuing my work in the acupuncture, herbal-medicine, and massage clinics, I asked medical colleagues to put me in contact with Qi Gong investigators in Beijing. The next week I was introduced to a Dr. Lu, who was an eighty-year-old doctor of traditional Chinese medicine, a massage expert, and a master of Qi Gong. Patients of Dr. Lu commonly felt terrific heat whenever Dr. Lu emitted Qi at them through his hands. I asked Dr. Lu to demonstrate this Oriental laying on of hands.

I lay down on an examination table in Dr. Lu's small clinic. The old doctor slowly positioned his hands over my stomach about six inches from my skin. I closed my eyes and waited for the heat. I felt nothing. I was disappointed. Dr. Lu, on the other hand, was not surprised.

"How much exercise do you get, Dr. Ai?"

At the time, I ran ten miles a day and did calisthenics with Tai Ji Quan every morning.

"And tell me about your eating and sleeping habits."

I told him that I had been eating mainly vegetables and rice for many months and that I was sleeping like a baby.

"Do you feel healthy?"

The truth was, I felt healthier than ever before in my life.

"I can see how healthy you are, Dr. Ai. It is to your credit that you have paid such attention to your living habits. But this also explains why you did not feel my Qi in the form of heat just now. You see, your own body's Qi is full and very strong. The amount that I could direct at you would be imperceptible, given your present state. If, on the other hand, you were in a weakened condition or very ill, then you would sense this heat without any question, I assure you."

By the summer of 1980, scientists in Beijing, Shanghai, and Sichuan had established official Qi Gong research laboratories. The most famous of these was the Qi Gong research unit affiliated with the Shanghai Institute of Traditional Chinese Medicine. I applied for a traveler's permit to go from Beijing to Shanghai. My Beijing medical instructors and official sponsors forwarded letters of introduction to the Shanghai medical authorities. I wanted to see a performance of psychokinesis in a government-sanctioned research laboratory.

En route to Shanghai I arranged for a clandestine meeting with the Qi Gong master who had moved the lantern for me months earlier. He traveled quite a distance to see me. He had unfortunately caught a severe upper-respiratory infection and laughed at how even Qi Gong masters get sick from time to time.

I asked the Qi Gong master to repeat his psychokinetic performance for me. He apologized, saying that he was too weak and feverish to attempt external Qi Gong. I coaxed him, and he reluctantly agreed to try.

I set up a weight on a string and suspended it from the ceiling of the room where I was staying. He attempted to move it from a yard away, as he had done with the lamp some months before. He failed. I was disappointed, and he was apologetic. We attributed the failure to temporary illness.

According to Chinese medical theory, his illness was caused by and consistent with his weakened Qi. From the theoretical standpoint, it should have been no surprise that he could not move the object. I apologized for having embarrassed him, and bid him farewell.

After I reached Shanghai, an American exchange scholar at Fudan University introduced me to a friend of his, a Shanghai doctor of Western medicine with considerable experience in Qi Gong. Because he asked to remain anonymous, I will refer to him as Dr. X.

Dr. X, who spoke impeccable English, had graduated from the Shanghai First Medical College in 1938 and received excellent training in Western medicine. He was a respected internist in one of Shanghai's finest hospitals.

In 1951, at age forty-one, Dr. X discovered he had high blood pressure (hypertension), with readings commonly as high as 180 over 130. By 1958, at age forty-eight, he had developed serious angina pectoris (coronary artery disease) as well as early signs of kidney failure. His blood pressure was often as high as 260 over 140. The Western medications he took for hypertension, heart problems, and kidney disease were not working. At this point he turned to the study of Qi Gong.

He had learned Qi Gong exercises as a young boy but never practiced them faithfully. He decided to study Qi Gong in earnest as a way of controlling his hypertension. In 1958 he joined an experimental group called the Qi Gong Hypertension Clinic, which consisted of Qi Gong experts from Shanghai and surrounding cities. The masters added to his understanding of the physical and meditative aspects of Qi Gong. By 1980 his blood pressure was normal (140 over 80), and he was taking no medications for heart or kidney disease. He firmly believed that Qi Gong exercises had radically improved his health.

He trusted Qi in spite of his Western training. He had personally seen Qi Gong masters move inanimate objects without touching them. He had experienced sensations of heat and pressure as a result of the manipulation of Qi. He was convinced that many serious illnesses could be treated with Qi Gong techniques. With his help, I was finally able to arrange a visit to the Qi Gong research unit of the Institute of Traditional Medicine—no small feat, given the veil of official secrecy usually thrown over its workings.

The Shanghai Institute of Traditional Chinese Medicine was housed in a severely imposing set of 1950s concrete buildings five miles from the center of Shanghai. At its entrance was a concrete archway decorated with huge, brass Chinese characters. These were a stunning, stylized calligraphy of the school's proud name. Below the arch stood my welcoming party, Dr. Lin Hai and Comrade Lin Ho-sheng.

Dr. Lin Hai, the director of the Qi Gong research unit, was a short, pensive man in his fifties with uncombable black hair projecting skyward as if pulled by static electricity. He, like most of the scientists I met, wore heavy, black-framed reading glasses with Coke-bottle-thick lenses. He had on standard attire—a white short-sleeved shirt, baggy blue cotton trousers, and plastic sandals.

Dr. Lin Hai shook my hand and introduced himself and his colleague, Comrade Lin Ho-sheng. Comrade Lin Ho-sheng was a Qi Gong master—not just any Qi Gong master, but the Qi Gong master shown on national television in the documentary that had caused a stir some months earlier. He was one of China's premier Qi Gong masters and the principal subject of study of the Qi Gong research unit.

Comrade Lin, also clad in white shirt, cotton trousers, and plastic sandals, was about forty. A short, powerfully built and soft-spoken man, he had large shoulders and a waist so small that his belt wrapped around twice. Like the other Qi Gong masters I had met, Lin possessed charisma that flowed equally from physical superiority and from emotional tranquillity.

Comrade Lin had practiced Qi Gong since the age of fifteen. During the Cultural Revolution he, like most other Qi Gong masters, did not perform or practice in public. Only in 1978, with the founding of the Qi Gong research unit, did he finally come forth. The research unit had no laboratory of its own and had to share equipment with the nearby nuclear-energy lab. The research unit boasted of some remarkable discoveries.

It claimed to have confirmed for the first time that Qi Gong masters could at will emit Qi from their fingertips. Researchers observed that when Qi Gong masters directed their Qi at sensing devices from a distance of one meter, energy waves could be detected. Director Lin Hai would not precisely define the type of energy emitted.

He reported that one could lower blood pressure not only by having patients practice Qi Gong exercises (e.g., internal Qi Gong) but also by having Qi Gong masters direct external Qi at acupuncture points of hypertensive patients. The distance between the Qi Gong master and the patient was roughly six to twelve inches. Director Lin and his colleagues said that systolic and diastolic blood pressure were lowered an average of 15 to 20 millimeters of mercury (e.g., from 160 over 100 to 140 over 80). They provided no published references.

Director Lin described how external Qi Gong had been used

to induce analgesia in patients undergoing surgery. Qi Gong masters like Lin Ho-sheng had been asked to focus their external Qi onto selected acupuncture points, where needles would otherwise have been inserted. I was given a photograph of Comrade Lin Ho-sheng gowned, gloved and masked, standing beside an operating table and aiming his fingers at acupuncture points on a patient's body. Director Lin Hai reported that twelve patients had undergone painless thyroidectomies and an additional three had had painless gastrectomies (removal of the stomach) with nothing more than 5 mg of Valium and Comrade Lin's external Qi for analgesia.

Both Director Lin Hai and Comrade Lin Ho-sheng knew how eager I was to see a demonstration. They agreed to show me an example of Lin Ho-sheng's talents. Comrade Lin closed the windows and shut off the electric fan in the room so that the air would be still. It was a brutally hot summer day, with temperatures between ninety and a hundred degrees. Comrade Lin took an ordinary piece of string attached to a needle and a two-centimeter-long piece of rubber with three feathers stuck into one end—a makeshift dart. He asked me to stick the needle into the dart and suspend it wherever I wished.

I tied the string to a latch at the top of the windowsill, about ten feet off the floor. The dart dangled in the air and twisted freely for a few seconds as we walked to the other end of the room to wait. In a minute the dart stopped moving. Lin put on a surgical face mask so that his breathing would not agitate the air as he approached the dart.

Comrade Lin carefully walked across the room, keeping his head and neck upright without swinging his arms. He could have been a cat stalking a bird; he was so silent and surefooted. As he got within a few feet of the dart, he brought his outstretched right arm into a horizontal position with his palm about three feet directly under the dart. He spread his fingers, and the muscles of his hand and forearm began to tremble slightly. Beads of sweat appeared on his forehead. His neck veins bulged as he took a deep breath and held it in for a moment. The dart remained motionless until Lin rotated his palm clockwise, at which time the dart rotated counterclockwise. When he held his hand absolutely still, the dart stopped moving. Sweating profusely, he repeated the twisting motion several times; each time the dart stopped or moved in synchrony with his hand. By bringing his left hand under the dart, he increased the rotation. Then, by moving his hands simultaneously in a horizontal plane, he set the dart swinging back and forth. He stepped back visibly fatigued, ripped the mask from his face, and yelled, "What do you think now?"

Like the experiment with the lantern months before, this demonstration *seemed* to suggest the existence of Qi. This time I had witnessed the phenomenon as an official guest of a government research laboratory.

Once Comrade Lin had rested enough to catch his breath, we talked again. I suggested that Qi Gong was an excellent topic for collaboration between East and West. Both Comrade Lin and Director Lin said they would be delighted to work with United States researchers. They admitted that they needed sophisticated equipment like nuclear magnetic resonance scanners and investigative know-how before they could proceed much further with their experiments. I told them that United States universities and parapsychology laboratories would quite likely want to share information related to Qi Gong and exceptional human body functions. They said they would be willing to go to the United States if such an exchange could be arranged.

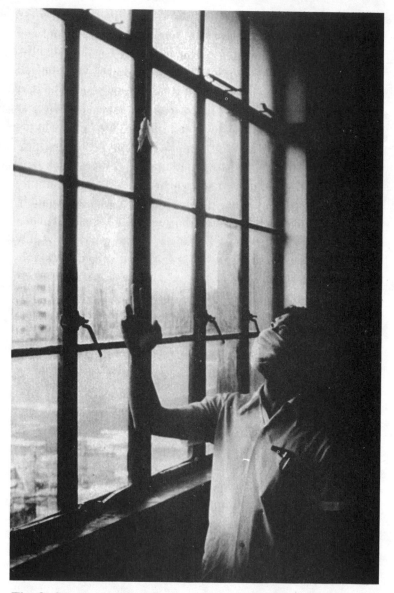

The Qi Gong master Lin Ho-sheng uses external Qi to move objects in the laboratories of the Shanghai Institute of Traditional Chinese Medicine.

"Yes, that would be a great honor," said the director. "We cannot expect to come up with all the answers in our small Shanghai research facilities."

"Have you discussed your work with many foreign doctors or scientists?"

"No," said Director Lin Hai. "You are the first foreign friend with whom we have discussed our research. You are also the first foreigner to see Comrade Lin Ho-sheng demonstrate his abilities. So you see, it has been a special day for us."

The Qi activities of the Chinese Qi Gong masters have parallels in phenomena found in other cultures. The Qi Gong master's alleged ability to move inanimate objects is not very different from the Indian yogi's alleged ability to levitate. Qi Gong investigations in telepathy resemble those conducted in parapsychology laboratories in the United States and the Soviet Union.* Accounts of Qi Gong masters' ability to heal are similar to tales of folk practitioners from many cultures throughout recorded history. What is lacking in all of these instances is proof— verifiable and reproducible proof that these phenomena do occur.

On the other hand, excessive skepticism can be as deleterious to scientific progress as excessive credulity. Aspects of Qi Gong practice may seem mysterious and unbelievable, yet there are historical precedents in Western medicine where equally unbelievable observations eventually gained acceptance. Imagine what it must have been like in the 1840s when ether anesthesia was introduced in America. The country general practitioner was

---

* Russell Targ and Keith Harary, *The Mind Race* (New York: Villard Books, 1984), and Sheila Ostrander and Lynn Schroeder, *Psychic Discoveries behind the Iron Curtain* (Englewood Cliffs: Prentice-Hall, 1970).

sure to doubt that Harvard Medical School eggheads, by merely soaking a cloth with some chemical (ether), had managed to induce a pain-free state that allowed patients to undergo major surgery without discomfort. It seemed unthinkable. Imagine what it was like in 1971 when, under the leadership of Dr. Paul Dudley White, a group of American scientists first witnessed acupuncture anesthesia and were confronted with the Chinese claim that sensations of pain could be stopped by the sticking of needles into flesh. It appeared preposterous but was true.

Practitioners and scholars of traditional Chinese medicine insisted that Qi is a physical as well as an intellectual entity. For 2,500 years China experimented with Qi as it related to the prevention of disease, the preservation of health, physical diagnosis, and the treatment of all human illnesses. In the 1970s in laboratories like the Shanghai research unit, modern Western scientific principles were applied to these experiments for the first time, and the preliminary findings were startling. But could these findings withstand the scrutiny of professional skeptics?

There was more to learn.

Dai-Fu:
"The Doctors"

Unlike doctors in the West, Chinese physicians are not wealthy and wield little social power. They are, to be sure, respected for their knowledge and dedication, but they earn less than factory workers. On the average a senior doctor takes home 59 to 115 yuan per month. That is equivalent to thirty to sixty United States dollars per month.*

The role of the classical Chinese physician, unlike that of most Western M.D.'s, was to teach patients to maximize health by living correctly. In many instances physicians were traditionally paid only as long as their patients remained in good health. When a patient became ill, fee payments stopped. The priority was clearly to prevent illness and maintain well-being. Only when prevention failed were therapeutic measures like acupunc-

---

* Dean Jamison et al., "China: The Health Sector," The World Bank, 1984.

ture or herbs used to restore bodily equilibrium.

The ideal physician in ancient China appreciated the superiority of prevention over intervention. Over two thousand years ago Chinese medical scholars wrote, "The sages did not treat those who were already ill; they instructed those who were not yet ill. To administer medicines to diseases which have already developed and to suppress the chaos which has already begun is comparable to the behavior of persons who begin to dig a well after they are thirsty and of those who begin to cast weapons after they are already engaged in battle. Would these actions not be too late? . . . The superior physician helps before the earliest budding of disease. . . . The inferior physician begins to help when the disease has already set in. And since his help comes when the disease has already developed, it is said of him that he is ignorant."*

According to traditional theory, health and longevity depend not only on environment, genetics, and fate but also on style of living, thoughts, and emotions. This view spawned a patient role drastically different from that of most modern medical consumers. The patient bore the primary responsibility for his or her health. Physicians did not *fix* broken bodies. They guided patients on personal quests for optimal physical and mental balance. This assistance came in the form of herbs, needles, massage, and, above all, recommendations for behavioral modification.

In this system physicians stood forth as role models of physical as well as mental discipline. In addition to being scholars, some physicians were also masters of the martial arts, especially the technique of Qi Gong. Exercise, viewed as an essential part of physical and mental health, was a high priority in imperial

---

* *The Yellow Emperor's Classic of Internal Medicine,* ca. third century B.C.

China and remains a high priority in modern China. Athletic classes are mandatory for university students. Each morning hundreds of millions of Chinese begin their day as their ancestors did—by exercising at dawn. Most perform Tai Ji Quan, and an increasing number are taking up Qi Gong. Some do calisthenics or jog. In every city, in every park, groups of people gather at 5:00 A.M. to perform the balletlike motion of Tai Ji Quan. To watch thousands of Chinese, many of them in their seventies or eighties, exercising in the dead of winter at sunrise is to witness a celebration of life—a reminder of the age-old maxim that life-style is an essential part of health.

While at Harvard Medical School I listened to countless lectures describing the complicated pathophysiology of disease. Sometimes I asked questions about the relation between diseases and life-style or psychological state. "We don't really know," one professor would say while presenting the latest research data on a particular disease. "There are no good studies available. Those which have been done are equivocal," another would say, referring to a different disease. Some faculty were less diplomatic: "Your questions are irrelevant to this discussion." My teachers' lack of interest in discussing the relation between one's life-style or mental state and the disease process was another example of the fundamental difference between the Chinese and Western medical systems.

The dichotomy of "traditional Chinese doctor" and "modern Western doctor" did not exist in China until the late nineteenth century, when Western medicine was formally introduced to the empire. American, European, and Japanese physicians established Western-style practices and built hospitals in the major cities of China. Fifty-six Western medical colleges existed in China before 1949. Some were run by state or provincial governments and others by missionaries or foreign organizations like

Harvard, Yale, St. John's University, and the Rockefeller Foundation. Graduates from these institutions were labeled "doctors of Western medicine" to distinguish them from doctors of traditional Chinese medicine.*

In the period from 1900 to 1949 Western medicine grew increasingly popular, particularly among the ruling class. At the same time leaders of traditional medicine and of Western medicine repeatedly denounced one another. Although most Chinese still preferred traditional medicine, the Nationalist government under Chiang Kai-shek passed legislation to outlaw traditional medicine on the grounds that it was backward and riddled with superstition. Traditional medical practices continued, however, and the majority of Chinese held on to their belief that traditional techniques were superior to those of Western medicine.

After the Communists came to power, in 1949, there was a shortage of Western-trained physicians. Only 38,000 doctors of Western medicine served a population of 500 million. The ratio of doctors to patients was 1 per 13,000 (compared with 1 per 500 in the United States at that time). But there were nearly 300,000 doctors of traditional medicine. Furthermore, traditional medicine was the preferred method of healing for the majority of the population.

At the First National Health Conference, in 1950, Chairman Mao Ze-dong called for the integration of Chinese and Western medicine: "Unite all medical workers young and old of the traditional and Western schools to organize a solid front. We must strive for the development of the people's health work."

---

* For a more complete discussion of the history of Western medicine in China, see Dean Jamison et al., "China: The Health Sector," The World Bank, 1984, and Mary Brown Bullock, *An American Transplant: The Rockefeller Foundation and Peking Union Medical College* (Berkeley: University of California Press, 1980).

Over the next fifteen years (1950 through 1965) the People's Republic of China took an idealistic and unconventional approach toward health care. It emphasized that medicine must serve the people—China's "peasants, workers, and soldiers." Preventive medicine received priority over interventional medicine. Major health problems, such as infectious diseases, were to be eradicated by means of massive public campaigns.

In 1965 the Cultural Revolution radically altered China's medical policy. During the chaotic years 1966–1971, all medical schools were closed. When they reopened, in 1972, medical curricula for schools of Western medicine and schools of traditional medicine were shortened from six years to three. One of those three years was to be spent in the countryside or in factories. Approximately one-third of the faculty of all medical schools and one-third of the staff of all urban hospitals were sent to the countryside with the objective of "making city dwellers aware of the peasant's life and problems, of keeping urbanites physically fit, and of promoting a sense of involvement at the grass-roots level."* Medical students were selected by the communities they served, on the basis not of academic performance but of motivation, ideology, and a dedication to "serve the people." The classical examination system was assailed by proponents of the Cultural Revolution, and all certification examinations were abolished. These extraordinary measures were consistent with the philosophy of the time (1972–1976), when it was far better to be "Red" than "expert."

In 1976, with the deaths of Zhou En-lai and Mao Ze-dong and with the overthrow of the infamous Gang of Four, the entire Chinese medical system was once again reexamined. A system

* T. O. Cheng et al., "Medical Education and Practice in the People's Republic of China," *Annals of Internal Medicine* 83 (1975): 716–24.

of entrance examinations was reestablished in 1977. Curricula were expanded from three years to five or six. In 1979 the Capital Hospital Medical College in Beijing began an eight-year training program that emphasized biomedical research. Traditional Chinese medical colleges were once again totally separated from Western-style medical colleges, and their curricula were lengthened to five or six years. The pendulum had swung back again.

Today one-fifth of China's medical students are enrolled in colleges of traditional Chinese medicine while the other four-fifths attend colleges of Western medicine. Doctors of Western medicine currently outnumber doctors of traditional medicine almost two to one.* Students of traditional medicine receive only minimal instruction in the basics of Western medical science; conversely, students at Western medical colleges graduate with no more than a rudimentary understanding of traditional Chinese medicine. According to data from the Ministry of Public Health, there are only 2,000 doctors with training in both traditional and Western medicine.†

These are the facts, figures, and policy changes that made their way into prestigious medical journals. But they fail to give a complete picture of China's medical workers. They do not tell the whole story of what life has been like for doctors in modern China.

During 1979 and 1980 I was a student of traditional Chinese medicine by day and a teacher of English by night. Three evenings a week, a black Russian-built sedan taxi met me at the gates

---

* The approximate numbers in 1982 were 303,000 doctors of traditional medicine and 557,000 doctors of Western medicine. See the *Statistical Yearbook of China* (Beijing: State Statistical Bureau, 1983).
† Dean Jamison et al., "China: The Health Sector," The World Bank, 1984, p. 143.

of the Beijing Institute of Traditional Chinese Medicine and dropped me off at either the Capital Hospital or the Beijing Second Medical College. These were Western-style medical centers staffed predominantly by doctors of Western medicine. I had volunteered to teach English to the faculty of both institutions. The two hundred physicians I met were eager to improve their conversational English. I was grateful for the opportunity to get to know these men and women personally and to share thoughts about life in our respective medical systems.

I gave my classes in an old lecture hall and in a run-down research laboratory where doctors sat in crowded rows of wooden desks. I stood before a chalkboard and behind a podium while reel-to-reel tape recorders (cassettes had not yet reached Beijing) captured every word. Our conversations ranged far and wide—over personal background, medicine, politics, daily life . . . you name it. For every class I prepared a talk on a specific aspect of medicine as it pertained to physicians in the United States, and in the next class the Chinese presented brief essays in English on facets of the physician's life and work in China. I corrected their grammar, spelling, and pronunciation, and they in turn helped me with my Chinese.

The first week of class, I delivered a long autobiographical sketch and asked the doctors to prepare their autobiographies for me.

Essay No. 1: *My Autobiography:*
"Fifty years ago, I was born in the beautiful city of Suzhou. . . . I graduated from the Shanghai Second Medical College, formerly known as the Medical College of St. John's University, in 1955. The name of the high school I graduated from was the Vincent Mille Academy of Suzhou.

"Before I went to primary school, my father began to teach

me English. But during the years of the Pacific Ocean war, I could learn only Japanese as Suzhou was overrun by the Japanese imperialists. I used my English in my medical training. Then, as was the custom in the early 1950s, I began to learn Russian.

"Before 1966, I worked and studied very hard and happily and followed the journals of the United States and the United Kingdom. I wrote articles about my own specialty. But all of these endeavors were considered faults to be harshly criticized under the control of the Gang of Four. This criticism led to great hardship.

"Although I like the arts, especially photography, I am now too busy to take up these hobbies, as I am learning English again, and I am also an editor of the *Beijing Medical Journal.* I always have a lot of things to do for my hospital.

"I write English very poorly since I have not had the chance to use it for thirty years.

"I am anxious to learn the modern knowledge from the USA and will be very grateful for your corrections indeed!"

Physicians who began medical school before liberation (1949) needed a working knowledge of English. They were taught medicine by American and European physicians who spoke no Chinese. Physicians fifty and older received excellent medical training and kept up with the international literature until the Cultural Revolution (1966), when they were criticized for being "intellectual elitists" who suffered from "Western influences." Most of these elder physicians were sent to the countryside for a period of "reeducation." Having survived the horrors of that era, these men and women regained positions of leadership and are currently redirecting China's Western medical system.

Autobiography No. 2: *Self-Introduction for Friendship*
"I was born in a factory worker's family in 1938. I am the
littlest child in our family. I learned Russian in the 1950s but
am self-taught in my English.
"I graduated from medical college in 1964. My specialty is
surgery. From 1970 to 1977 during the mid-stage of the great
Cultural Revolution, I was sent to a commune hospital in the
northwest countryside. Medical students were also sent. This
was called 'the integration between serving and studying.' I was
the head of our little hospital located in a mountain region.
"My purpose for being there was to reeducate and serve the
poor and lower-middle peasants. Life there was very difficult,
and the people worked very hard. Before we went there, the
hygiene of the people was poor and many died. There were no
doctors there to treat them, so people often looked to medicine
men or witches.
"After we came to know the miserable conditions of the
region, my companions and I decided to overcome our difficulties. We established an operating room, bought or borrowed
equipment, and saved hundreds of patients.
"We also organized a mobile medical team to make rounds on
patients who could not go to the hospital. We traveled every day
to one house after another. Sometimes we could only see one or
two patients each day. We propagated hygienic knowledge,
trained the barefoot doctors, and carried out birth control and
preventive inoculations. Because of our works, we won praise
and respect from the masses.
"Of course, in the ten-year catastrophe of the Cultural Revolution, Chinese intellectuals (and this includes doctors) had a very
low position in society. Too much time was wasted.
"But I think that adverse circumstances are the best exercises
for a person. And so it is to me."

Physicians in their forties attended medical school during the 1950s, an era when relations between China and the Soviet Union were at their best. These physicians learned Russian but not English. Their preliminary medical education was sound, but their advanced training suffered considerably because of their reassignment during the Cultural Revolution.

Autobiography No. 3: *Name: Cai Hong, Age: 29*

"I graduated from middle school in 1967. Because of the Cultural Revolution, I was deprived of the opportunity to further my studies and went to work on a farm in Heilongjiang Province, northeast of Mongolia. I was only sixteen years old, and although the manual labor was interesting and I was in excellent health, it was unfortunate that I was not allowed to study.

"After working on the farm for four and a half years, I went to work in a hospital as a laborer. This hospital had been built for oil workers.

"Fortunately, in 1976 a training class in medicine was established. It was different from a true medical college. For example, work in the hospital was considered more important than studying textbooks and the duration of school courses was shorter than conventional medical college.

"I started learning to be a doctor. We studied preclinical courses but only for a short period of eight months. After that we learned and worked for three months in clinical medicine and surgery, one and one half months in pediatrics and gynecology, and two weeks only in ophthalmology, otolaryngology, and dermatology.

"In addition, we all went to Mt. Tang to help victims of a natural calamity—a great earthquake.

"After two years of study, I graduated and was appointed to work as an intern in the department of medicine for one year.

Because my knowledge of basic science was poor, I wanted to study it deeper. I prepared for the national postgraduate examination and did my best to get an excellent mark. I was glad that I passed, and since October 1979 I have been a postgraduate student.

"My specialty is biochemistry. My task of study is the nucleic acid metabolism and protein synthesis of cancer. My greatest interest is in molecular biology. I have little professional experience because of my background."

The youngest generation of Chinese doctors, those now in their thirties, studied medicine during the most tumultuous years of modern China. Their education was fragmented from beginning to end. Their last years in secondary school were disrupted because of the initial turmoil of the Cultural Revolution. The select few who were granted an opportunity to study medicine did so in commune clinics or in factory hospitals, learning whatever they could from mobile medical teams and precious medical texts. Thousands of these doctors spent five to ten years in the countryside performing physical labor while contending with a complex, constantly changing political hierarchy. Those who learned English studied it on their own through books and occasional English-language radio broadcasts.

What sets this youngest generation of doctors apart from those in their forties, fifties, and sixties is not the high degree of personal suffering but the inadequacy of their medical training. With no more than two or three years of formal medical education, these men and women were expected to perform like competent clinicians. Even the most industrious and dedicated, Cai Hong among them, could not master all of medicine in two years.

Since 1979 these younger physicians have been encouraged to attend "postgraduate" training programs. The term *postgradu-*

ate is a bit of a euphemism. These younger doctors are indeed "graduates," but they are the first to admit that their medical education has been inadequate, and they are eager to "restudy" medical basics, which they never fully mastered. Those who pass a qualifying examination will have this opportunity in a series of custom-tailored "postgraduate training programs."

Autobiography No. 4: *The Barefoot Doctor*
"My name is Sun Li-zhe. I am twenty-eight years old. I graduated from a junior middle school attached to Xin Hua University in 1967. After graduation I went to the countryside as an 'educated youth.' I was sixteen. I lived and worked in the Yenan Mountains for ten years.

"The second year after my arrival I was selected as a barefoot doctor by the local villagers. I had to learn medical knowledge and skills in a self-taught way.

"I was trained but only for three months by a People's Liberation Army medical team. With the help of the local peasants and other barefoot doctors, we set up a cooperative medical clinic and treated a number of diseases.

"Last year I was accepted by the Beijing Second Medical College as a postgraduate student. My specialty is surgery of the liver, gall bladder, and pancreas."

Sun Li-zhe, who became one of my closest friends, was being modest in this initial autobiographical essay. He is in fact something of a modern Chinese hero.

After being chosen the local "barefoot doctor" in the mountains of northwest China, the eighteen-year-old Sun Li-zhe was given a copy of the *Barefoot Doctor's Manual,* a few needles, and a few herbs; so armed, he was expected to deliver primary medical care to the masses.

Sun Li-zhe realized that his self-taught medical skills were inadequate. Acutely ill patients in need of surgical intervention (especially those suffering from gall stones or appendicitis) died before they could reach the nearest hospital. Sun Li-zhe took it upon himself to do something about this calamity. He acquired several surgical textbooks and studied them diligently.

He then attempted abdominal operations on dogs, pigs, and chickens. His materials were makeshift, his operating conditions primitive. After much preparation Sun Li-zhe performed his first operation on a patient. With the equivalent of only a high school education and three months of formal medical training, Sun Li-zhe removed the appendix of an acutely ill woman and saved her life. During the ten years that Sun Li-zhe lived in Yenan, he performed more than one hundred major abdominal operations, incurred no serious complications, and saved many lives. His professional skill and his irrepressible desire to "serve the people" earned him national acclaim.

Like Cai Hong, Sun Li-zhe taught himself English and prepared for the rigorous entrance examinations that would allow him to return to Beijing as a "postgraduate student." He passed these examinations at such a high level that he was permitted to enroll as a postgraduate trainee without ever having actually attended medical school.

Sun Li-zhe is currently an exchange student living in the United States and studying advanced immunology. He hopes someday to realize a lifelong dream by working as a transplant surgeon in Beijing.

The motivation of young people who become physicians is a complicated subject. For some doctors in China and the West, the answer is simple: overt family pressure.

Autobiography No. 5: *"Why I am a Doctor"*
"You asked in your last class what it is that makes people want to become a doctor. My father is a doctor. His father is a doctor. My mother is a nurse. My younger brother is a doctor of traditional medicine. My bigger younger sister is a doctor, my little younger sister is a nurse, my wife is a pediatrician, and my brother-in-law is a doctor too! Everyone in my family except my oldest brother is a doctor or a nurse. For me to study medicine is an easy decision."

The physicians in my English classes were surprised to learn that American M.D.'s have the freedom to select whatever specialty they choose and to set up practice wherever they like. In China such decisions rest on complicated quota systems established by national plenary commissions. The final, nitty-gritty decisions as to which medical graduates are assigned to which specialties and where each will be sent to work are made by special committees of political leaders and medical personnel. When I asked the doctors in my classes for details about who sat on these powerful committees and how they reached their decisions, I was told, "We don't honestly know those details. Our political leaders know, but we are not told."

In time the doctors in my English classes became my friends. It is rare for Chinese to invite foreign guests into their apartments. Most feel that their living conditions are too poor to serve as a suitable place for entertainment of this kind. After a couple of months, my new friends put aside their pride and invited me in.

The physicians' apartments were akin to inner-city tenements, tiny one- or two-bedroom flats, most without a private bathroom. A desktop doubled as a cooking surface, the bedroom was also the sitting room, and the kitchen was smaller than an American closet. Physicians owned bicycles but no cars. Like everyone else in China, they needed ration coupons to buy rice or cotton garments.

The living conditions of my physician friends emphasize yet another difference between medicine as it is practiced in China and in the West. In America students appear at their medical school interviews gushing with altruism. "I want to help people; I want to direct my interests in science toward skills which will help others; I like working with people and want to help." These words are spoken with the deepest conviction. Unfortunately, during eight or ten or fifteen years of training, many American doctors grow callous and lose their passion for helping others. They are seduced by wealth or status or prestige, or they are just too exhausted to continue caring. For Chinese doctors, however, there is no room for a change of heart. Neither wealth nor status nor power is guaranteed with the job. If Chinese doctors lose sight of their love for medicine or their desire to be of service to others, then they are left with nothing.

Happily, there is no shortage of life's simpler pleasures in China. My doctor friends invited me to spend weekends with them cooking, lingering in museums, or taking long walks around the Forbidden City or the Summer Palace. Sun Li-zhe, the famous barefoot doctor, was a fishing addict and called me weekly to go fishing with him.

A typical expedition with Sun Li-zhe began at 6:30 A.M. at the front gates of Beijing University. He would be waiting there on his bicycle wearing his wrinkled navy-blue Mao jacket and matching pants, carrying his barefoot doctor's pack jammed with food and bait and extra tackle. His crew cut was always in need of a trim, his thick glasses listed to one side, and his body was in perpetual motion. Blessed with the energy of ten men and known to be as mischievous as ten children, Sun Li-zhe was ever prepared for fun.

We would bike together to the Summer Palace and make our way toward the reservoir behind the lake. In April the magnolia trees were in full bloom. By seven in the morning there were already tens of thousands of visitors who had come to enjoy the magnificent flowers. We would push our way past the palace grounds and walk beyond the famous marble boat and water lily ponds. Crossing a small bridge, we would come to the reservoir that Sun Li-zhe knew to be the best fishing spot.

Along the water's edge for a mile or more sat dozens of solitary fishermen separated from one another by twenty or thirty yards. Each had two or three homemade fishing rods prepared from bamboo poles attached to string. There were a couple of primitive spinning reels—handmade, of course. The fishermen put a bit of cornmeal on their hooks, cast out their lines, then stuck the butt of their rods in the ground, put their hands in their pockets, and waited. It was peaceful by that reservoir. No radios blaring, no beer cans popping, just silence and the smell of springtime.

Unlike the other fishermen, Sun Li-zhe approached fishing with the indomitable zeal he applied to medicine. He changed bait every five minutes, maneuvered his poles every which way, and paced the waterfront inspecting other people's catches. I had asked my family to send me, as a gift for Sun Li-zhe, an American fishing rod and reel. When I handed it to him, he cradled it in his hands as if he were holding the crown jewels of London and said "Oh, this is the most beautiful gift in the world. I don't know what to say." Then his devilish humor emerged: "There is one horrible thing about this gift, though. I'm afraid I may have a relapse of the dreaded fishing sickness."

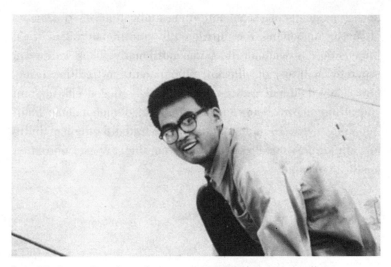

Sun Li-zhe, a barefoot doctor with "fishing sickness."

"Fishing sickness?" I asked. "Yes. Years ago, while I was in the mountains of Yenan, I never told you this, but I was stricken with the fishing sickness. Whenever I was sick my mind was filled only with thoughts of fishing and nothing else. It is a very serious condition, and the symptoms can be very severe. There is no cure. This rod and reel may weaken me. I may have a relapse. Well, I will try not to blame you, as you did not know of my illness."

Many a weekend Sun Li-zhe and I sat on the banks of that Beijing reservoir, casting out cornmeal with one fiberglass rod and three Stone Age poles. We drank plum wine and ruminated about medicine on our opposite sides of the globe.

To my surprise, Sun Li-zhe and other doctors of Western medicine seldom had contact with doctors of traditional medicine. Western-style physicians sent to the countryside saw traditional medicine firsthand, but they rarely used acupuncture, herbal medicine, massage, and other applications of Qi. Doctors of Western medicine were intrigued by traditional practices, yet they could not condone them unconditionally. They worked in separate facilities and did not refer patients to traditional doctors. They doubted traditional medicine's alleged efficacy and voiced skepticism about reports of Qi-related phenomena. Traditional doctors were understandably frustrated by their inability to gain professional recognition from their Western-oriented medical colleagues.

On
Mental Illness:
"Freud's
Not Here"

The array of psychopathology that exists in the West also exists in China. Types of mental disorders, including their subtypes, have been identified among the Chinese using standard Western diagnostic criteria.* Psychiatric disturbances are common to East and West, but there are radical differences in the ways they are perceived, interpreted, and treated.

Traditional Chinese doctors apply a single conceptual mode to both physical and mental illness. In this framework, mental well-being influences and is influenced by all other bodily functions. An imbalance of emotions can disturb the function of internal organs and vice versa. An excess of happiness is said

---

* Arthur Kleinman and Tsung-yi Lin, eds., *Normal and Abnormal Behavior in Chinese Culture* (Dordrecht: D. Reidel, 1981).

to damage the "heart"; anger, the "liver"; worry, the "lung"; fear, the "kidney"; and desire, the "spleen." There is no separation of mind from body. They are interdependent and in a constant state of change. This is an extension of the principle of Yin and Yang as applied to mental health.

Mental well-being is said to exist when there is a "balanced state," a harmony of Yin and Yang. A patient's physical state can be judged in terms of symptoms or pulse and tongue diagnosis, but how is one to judge a patient's mental state? In its approach to this question, too, Chinese medicine has borrowed from Chinese philosophy.

To achieve a "balanced mental state," one traditionally had to live according to prescribed virtues. These included filial piety, a respect for one's elders, an appreciation for nature, a keen sense of moral obligation, loyalty, self-governance, self-denial, privacy, moderation, and an inhibition of outward emotion. These virtues, most of them Confucian in origin, helped to define a balanced state, the mind at peace. Such a mind ensured bodily health, and bodily health ensured a mind at peace.

A severely "imbalanced mental state," as manifested by retardation, psychosis, or suicide, was attributed to defective Qi. This defective Qi was felt to have been inherited ("congenital Qi") and was attributed to flaws in one's ancestors or "bad spirits" afflicting one's ancestral line. Mental illness thus became a cause for shame, a curse on an entire household.

Small wonder, then, that Chinese attempted wherever possible to deny mental illness by ascribing emotional or psychological disturbance to a physical problem. They attributed emotional pain or psychological abnormality to an imbalance in some internal organ and not to a primary mental illness. This process is known as somatization. In all but the most disturbed patients (the frankly psychotic, for example), it offered an acceptable

170

explanatory model for abnormal behavior or dysphoria. It relieved the burden of guilt associated with the designation "mental illness." Somatization is not unique to China, of course, but it is pervasive there.

Three of China's most commonly used psychiatric labels are neurasthenia *(shen jing shuai ruo)*, hysteria *(yi bing)*, and schizophrenia *(jing shen fen lie)*. The vast majority of China's doctors, both modern and traditional, have not studied any psychiatry and are not familiar with standardized psychiatric criteria for making diagnoses. Chinese patients labeled "hysterical" or "schizophrenic" do not conform to any standard Western diagnostic criteria. *Shen jing shuai ruo* (neurasthenia) literally means "a weakening in the channels of the spirit." The textbook used at the Beijing Institute of Traditional Chinese Medicine* defined *neurasthenia* as "a functional disturbance of the central nervous system caused by a temporary imbalance of higher center activity induced by mental factors. . . . Symptoms vary, but the main ones include insomnia, fatigue, anxiety and depression. . . . If the patient complains of the above symptoms, yet no organic pathological changes are found upon physical examination, then neurasthenia can be diagnosed." According to traditional medical theory, neurasthenia is attributed to a weakness or disruption of Qi, in the "heart," "liver," "spleen," or "kidney." Treatment aims at "calming the spirit of the 'heart,' " strengthening the "kidneys," and regulating the "liver" and "spleen."

Neurasthenia, which does not exist as an acceptable diagnosis in Western psychiatry, is the quintessential example of somatization. The attribution of almost any emotional or psychological complaint to "neurasthenia" unburdens the patient from social

---

* *An Outline of Chinese Acupuncture* (Beijing: Foreign Languages Press, 1975).

stigma. His or her problem is then seen as a physical malady and not a mental disorder. The term *neurasthenia* is applied idiosyncratically to a range of minor mental disorders, including depression, anxiety, hypochondria, and hysteria.

Between one-third and one-half of the patients I saw in the Dong Zhi Men acupuncture, herbal medicine, and massage clinics admitted to "suffering from neurasthenia." In the West these patients would have been reclassified as suffering from depression or some anxiety disorder. This may at first seem like an extraordinarily high proportion. However, a similar fraction of Western patients have psychological or functional complaints—that is, complaints for which their doctor finds no apparent organic cause.

With somatization comes the expectation on the part of the patient that his or her problem will be amenable to some medicament, say, a pill or an herbal tea or an injection. Neurasthenics who are anxious or depressed or unable to sleep want a quick remedy that will reestablish bodily harmony and quell their symptoms. Sometimes these patients will accept as sole treatment the suggestion of a life-style or attitudinal change. More often than not, however, they anticipate at least some medication or acupuncture. These Chinese patients are not so very different from American clinic patients.

The greatest difference between East and West in the area of mental health has to do with the patient's willingness to communicate personal problems to a physician. There is a proverb in Chinese that says, *"Jia chou bu ke wai yang"* ("Domestic problems must not become public shame"). Whereas the uninhibited expression of personal problems to a therapist or doctor is accepted in the West, it is taboo in China. The Chinese are culturally disinclined to "talk out" their problem with a stranger—

even if that stranger is their physician. Chinese doctors are very sensitive to their patients' privacy and pride. These physicians are far more reluctant than even a reticent Westerner to pry into the psychosocial or sexual histories of their patients.

The Student

One morning a handsome young man in a smart blue jacket walked into our acupuncture clinic, went directly to the back of the room, and sat down on a treatment table. Dr. Zhang knew the boy's history in detail.

"He's eighteen years old," said Dr. Zhang. "A high school student. He is hysterical."

"How do you know?"

"Well, he's been out of school since last autumn. He comes here regularly for treatments."

"But why?"

"Because he is hysterical. The boy can no longer understand anything he reads. He used to be an excellent student. But now his brains are jumbled."

"What else can you tell me?"

"Well, the boy's behavior is odd. Every morning he gets up at dawn, exercises excessively, does Tai Ji Quan, and takes a shower. If he doesn't exercise rigorously every morning and bathe twice a day, he complains that he feels uncomfortable. Sometimes he even repeats this routine at night. When he cannot exercise according to his own rigid schedule, he complains more." Dr. Zhang walked over and took the boy's pulse. "He suffers from what is called 'excessive and rebellious Qi.' With such an imbalance the 'heart' cannot remain calm, and the spirit becomes unsettled." Zhang inserted two-inch needles into the boy's forehead, cheeks, scalp, arms, and legs. He used points on six different acupuncture meridians. When the boy opened his mouth, the needles surrounding his lips flowed back and forth in waves.

I walked over to his examining table. Trying to put him at ease, I spoke of our mutual interest in running and in Tai Ji Quan. After describing his exercise routine, he asked me what it was like to run a marathon. He wanted to do that someday.

"What about this reading problem of yours?" I asked.

"About a year and a half ago, I was transferred to a special high school for excellent students. All of my colleagues were preparing for the university entrance examination. After a few months, the work got more and more difficult. I fell behind in my classes. The teacher thought I was ill. He told my father."

The boy's father, I learned from Dr. Zhang, was a Western-style surgeon and medical director of a factory hospital. He had taken his son to three Beijing hospitals for an evaluation of his problem. The doctors at these hospitals had not been trained formally in psychiatry and had little experience with psychiatric patients. They told the boy that he had hysteria or perhaps schizophrenia. They offered no cure for either disease and suggested he go to the Institute of Traditional Chinese Medicine for treatment.

The boy's mother had gone to university before liberation (1949). She had been a science teacher but stopped teaching soon after the boy's birth. "My mother has been sick ever since she gave birth to me. Nobody is certain exactly what disease she has. She's tired a good deal and rarely goes out of the house. She thinks it's caused by neurasthenia. . . ."

"Do you have any brothers or sisters?"

"Yes. I have an older sister."

"How is she?"

"She has excellent health, is a first-rate student and has already enrolled at university. She makes my family very proud. . . ."

"I imagine your parents want you to go to university very badly."

"Yes. But they never talk to me about it."

"Do you think there is anything really wrong with you?"

There was a pause as the boy stared at the wall. The needles stopped quivering. He looked up and quietly said, "No."

This young man had been examined at three Western hospitals in Beijing, none of which had a department of psychiatry or a fully trained psychiatrist. Nonetheless, his hand-held medical record book carried the label "hysteric/schizophrenic."

The psychological pressures of academic performance are not unique to Chinese students. However, in China where an estimated 500 million people are under the age of thirty, the competition for a university education is unparalleled. In years past, admission to a Chinese university depended not only on examinations but also on recommendations of peers and political superiors. Today the examination is everything. Those who score in the top 4 percent will receive a formal education and find excellent jobs. The remaining 96 percent must accept the work they are assigned to do. This frequently means waiting for months or years following graduation from high school. Fear of academic failure among teenagers, particularly those from professional families, often reaches pathological proportion.

From an orthodox Western medical standpoint the boy in the Dong Zhi Men clinic needed psychotherapy. Instead, he received needles three times a week. I do not know his progress.

The Soldier

A soldier came into our massage clinic wearing army fatigues, matching polyester socks, and brown plastic sandals. His hair was crew cut and his chin had a stubble of beard. His arms hung at his sides like lead rods. He walked stooped over and forced his right arm to move forward with his right leg. Even as he sat down, his motions were awkwardly rigid. His main complaint: stiff shoulders.

Examining his strong upper back and large shoulders, I could not discern the normal landmarks of anatomy. His muscles and tendons felt like hardened rubber. When I asked what troubled him, he would just say, "I'm stiff, that's all. My body is stiff."

With time, massage, exercise, and acupressure, he began to regain movement of his shoulders and arms. But his manner remained unchanged. He showed no emotion, and his face was expressionless.

"I don't understand his condition," I said to Dr. Sun Shu, my massage instructor. "Can you tell me about him?"

Dr. Sun grew reflective. We went into the next room to be out of earshot of the other patients. "This soldier has had a most unfortunate life. He was an aide to General Lin Biao, who at one point was Chairman Mao's handpicked successor. But Lin Biao became involved in a plot to overthrow Chairman Mao and ultimately died in a mysterious plane crash. Lin Biao was branded an archenemy of the people. Until a few weeks ago this soldier had been in prison for nine years. He lived in solitary confinement, often in a cell the size of half a man, and was made to do harsh physical labor. His wife denounced him and divorced him during the Cultural Revolution. His family and friends abandoned him. His heart has known much bitterness these past nine years. This should tell you why his body is stiff and his consciousness dulled."

"What was his crime?" I asked.

"Nothing, Dr. Ai. Nothing. No formal charges were ever brought against him. He was an attendant to the wrong powerful person at the wrong time. During the years of the Cultural Revolution, there were many like him. Too many. They suffered more than you can know. Some came to our massage clinic after years in prison with their hands crossed at the wrists. They were in the habit of being shackled night and day, and after their release they asked our massage doctors to relieve their bodies of this habitual malady. Some had to learn to move all over again. They are a pitiful part of our national shame. The bodies of these prisoners, like the spirit of China, suffered greatly during the Cultural Revolution. It is terrible. Terrible."

The soldier had been publicly "rehabilitated," given nine years of back pay, and released from prison. Since his release the doctors in our clinic had become his closest acquaintances.

I paid special attention to the soldier and wanted to draw him out of his shell, to get him to relax and talk more in the presence of others. He was quite understandably withdrawn and depressed.

The other doctors did not give him undue attention. They feared the soldier would misconstrue public notice as pity and become even more withdrawn. They reminded me of the proverb "Personal problems must not become public shame."

While kneading his shoulder muscles, rubbing his neck, and rotating his joints, I talked with the soldier and assured him he was making great progress. Now and then I would press an acupuncture point near his armpit or foot and try to tickle him, hoping to arouse a smile.

"Make small progress day by day," another proverb says. That is what the soldier did. After a month of treatment, his muscles and tendons loosened. He was smiling spontaneously. He said "Good morning" without being spoken to. He was reentering the world of normalcy, working his way out of a deep depression.

This patient's life and psyche were scarred by the events of the Cultural Revolution (1965–1976). The chaos of that decade placed a unique psychological stress on tens of millions of Chinese. Intellectuals and professionals were separated from their families and sent into the countryside to plant rice or to perform menial tasks. The theory was that work in the fields would foster solidarity with the masses. In that era it was a crime to be an intellectual, to have overseas relations, or to come from a wealthy family.

A physician described the atmosphere of the Cultural Revolution as follows: "Under the rule of the Gang of Four, a person would lose his freedom suddenly. He would be examined—his history, point of view, overseas relations—and he would be criticized at mass meetings. Everyone was there. If he or his family could not accept this, they would be said to have a mental disorder."

The present government is trying to undo the ten years of psychological stress brought about during the Cultural Revolution. It is trying to make a fresh start, to modernize the state, and to rehabilitate those who suffered under the Gang of Four. However, the psychic scars of the Cultural Revolution remain an enormous problem for the Chinese people. This problem will require a good deal of medical attention in the years ahead. Leaving this work to practitioners of acupuncture, massage, and herbal medicine will not be sufficient. A generation of psychologists and psychiatrists is desperately needed in China.

The Mechanic

A patient in his early twenties came into our herbal-medicine clinic and handed his identification papers and medical booklet to Dr. Weng.

The patient was a driver and car mechanic for the Beijing Second Medical College. He wore baggy, gray cotton pants, black cotton shoes, and a plain white shirt and carried a blue Mao hat. He had acne and the hint of a mustache. With head bowed and his cap on his lap, he muttered, "I have neurasthenia, and I would like some medicines." His symptoms: insomnia, fatigue, an inability to concentrate. He denied having had any serious illnesses in the past. Avoiding eye contact, he spoke only when spoken to and conveyed a deep sadness.

Dr. Weng tapped on the desktop, and the young man presented his wrist for examination. "Pulse, thready and quick," wrote Dr. Weng with his fine quill pen in the man's cardboard medical book.

"Show me your tongue." It was pale, enlarged, and uncoated. There were dental indentations on its edges. The pulse and tongue diagnosis suggested a deficiency of Qi in his "heart" and "kidneys."

Dr. Weng told the young man not to worry. Some herbal medications would greatly improve him. Weng reached for his prescription pad and in bold calligraphy wrote the names of ten herbal medications.

I then broke the rules of standard Chinese medical decorum. Because I suspected that this man was severely depressed but unwilling to admit it, I did what I usually do with such patients. I began to ask rather personal questions in an effort to understand the patient's condition and enable him to ventilate his feelings a bit. In my own training this process had been called a "psychological incision and drainage procedure."

"Can you tell me if you've been experiencing any personal problems that might be influencing your neurasthenia?"

"No. Everything is fine," he said, staring at his shoelaces and picking lint off his socks.

"Tell me about your work. How has it been going?"

"It's not very hard. I like working with cars."

"How about your family?"

"Fine."

"How about your friends? Have you been having any problems with close friends lately?"

There was a silence that he punctuated with a deep sigh. Then the young man looked up from the floor. His eyes were glazed. "There is one thing," the man said. "Last week my fiancée was stabbed to death by a stranger in the street."

Dr. Weng lifted his head and put down his quill pen. He stared at the young patient but said nothing. He, too, had gathered that the young man was emotionally troubled but did not know to what extent. He chose not to ask prying questions. Nor did he ask for any gruesome details about the young man's fiancée. Dr. Weng pursed his lips and shook his head from side to side. Where in the view of a physician whose philosophy of medicine and life is based on balances and harmonies, I wondered, was there a place for senseless violence and murder? Weng rewrote his prescription, this time adding four potent sedatives to the mixture of herbal remedies.

The Woman with the Crooked Jaw

In the acupuncture clinic, a forty-five-year-old overweight woman pushed her way past the other patients to fight for the stool by Dr. Zhang's desk. She wore five layers of clothing even though it was a warm spring day. Because her nose was stuffed, she breathed through her mouth in a course, phlegmy way that might drive you mad if you sat alone with her in a quiet room. She was sweating, her gray trousers were too short, and her bright-red·thermal underwear dangled below her pant cuffs draped over her sagging malodorous socks.

Dr. Zhang asked the first question, "What is your problem?"

"I am hysterical," the woman said, snorting an audible puff of air through her clogged nose.

Dr. Zhang was unimpressed as the woman huffed and puffed like a child on the verge of an asthmatic fit. "Look at my mouth," she said. "It's not right. My jaw is crooked."

A textbook of traditional Chinese medicine describes hysteria as follows: "It includes complicated and variable clinical manifestations like sensory and motor disturbance, paralysis, sensory loss, aphasia, blindness and deafness. There may be emotional disturbances with unmotivated crying or laughing, constant movement and restlessness. These symptoms do not correspond with the results of physical examination."*

Zhang and I studied the woman's facial features. When she was at rest, her lower jaw jutted off to one side. When she spoke, it did not deviate from its proper position. When she drank a cup of water or smoked a cigarette (uncommon for a Chinese woman), there was no malalignment whatsoever.

"It's just when I'm not talking or eating that there's a problem. My friends noticed it yesterday and suggested I come to visit you. I didn't want to, but they said I should. I think I'm hysterical. Would you needle me, please?"

"What other diseases have you had in the past?" asked Dr. Zhang.

"Well, I've been hysterical many times before, and I've suf-

* *An Outline of Chinese Acupuncture* (Beijing: Foreign Languages Press, 1975).

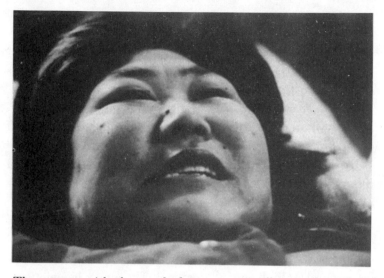

The woman with the crooked jaw: treating "neurasthenia" with acupuncture.

fered from neurasthenia for fifteen years. It all started with the Gang of Four and the Cultural Revolution. I'm quite certain it's hysteria this time and not just my neurasthenia. Can you fix it? Which table should I lie down on?"

Dr. Zhang pointed to a treatment table and went to the far end of the room to select his needles. The woman removed her winter coat, padded jacket, sweater, and cotton shirt, leaving on just a T-shirt. Dr. Zhang began placing needles in her arms and face. He felt for the appropriate points, rubbed them with alcohol, and inserted the needles effortlessly. The woman showed no signs of pain, telling Dr. Zhang that she had "obtained the Qi" with each needle insertion. She described a generalized fullness in the needled areas. When Zhang finished placing the needles, he went to minister to another patient. I asked some questions of my own.

"In my country, we often ask our patients to tell us something about themselves in order to understand their medical condition. Would you tell me a little about yourself, your family, your work, and living arrangements?"

The woman did not answer. I knew that I was on shaky ground asking such questions. She sat there with a dozen needles coming out of her face, neck, and ears. I could not tell whether I had said the wrong thing. I repeated my question clearly.

"I don't work," the woman said. "I have never worked. If I had gone to work, then I could have barely earned enough money to pay for a baby-sitter to watch the children. So I didn't work and stayed home to care for the children myself. Now I am becoming old. I suffer from neurasthenia. And I have no health insurance, because I never worked."

Health insurance programs are offered only to those employed by the state or communes.

"Tell me about your husband."

"He hasn't lived with me since 1966. That was the start of the Cultural Revolution. They said he was needed in the countryside in Hunan Province to be a welder for the army. My neurasthenia started then. My husband was finally relocated to Beijing last fall. But he has no job yet."

"What about your children?"

"Well, the two older boys are good at making trouble and nothing else. They have not found work since high school graduation. It's been more than a year that each has waited for work. My youngest one is a good student. But he can't make up for the others."

"Tell me," I said, "do you think any of your medical problems like your neurasthenia or hysteria could be related to the difficulties you've had with your family situation?"

"No," she said immediately. "What does family have to do with a nerve disease?"

This was a typical reaction for a patient carrying the label "neurasthenic." She had been given this label because of her insomnia, fatigue, and anxiety. She viewed her problem as a physical one, a malady related to her "nerves" rather than to her mind. She was not ashamed of her "nerve condition" and blamed it entirely on the Cultural Revolution. She spoke freely of her diagnosis, as if proud in some peculiar way that she had survived the horrors of the Cultural Revolution and as if her neurasthenia were proof of her suffering. In China there are many patients like this with chronic anxiety or depression who are labeled neurasthenics. Lacking insight into the personal and social stresses that influence their condition, they generally somatize their problems. The exact numbers are undocumented, but many seek the advice of traditional doctors and ask them to "fix their nerves" with a combination of acupuncture and herbs. There have been no prospective clinical trials testing the efficacy of these treatments.

Young Women and Childbearing

A twenty-four year-old woman arrived at the herbal-medicine clinic wearing a blue Mao jacket, blue pants, a white blouse buttoned to the top, white socks that had doily-like lace frills, and a pair of shiny black plastic sandals. She had freckles and pigtails, was pigeon-toed, and looked like a teenager, though she was considerably older.

"You have what illness?" asked Dr. Weng.

"My head feels light. I am dizzy. I sleep poorly."

"For how long?"

"Three months," answered the young woman.

184

"Do you have any other illnesses?"

"No."

Dr. Weng tapped the table with his fingers, and the woman placed her wrists alongside his hands. The woman began to blush. She was sitting bolt upright, her fists clenched so tightly that her knuckles were white. While keeping her knees together, she turned her ankles so that they were more pigeon-toed than ever.

"Perhaps I should tell you. I've been trying to have a baby but I'm not pregnant yet."

"Oh," said Dr. Weng. "When did you marry?"

"Three months ago, when I became twenty-four. My husband and I want to have a child. We have dreamed of having a child since we first decided to marry nine years ago. We got married as soon as we were old enough [legal age in China for marriage was twenty-four for women and twenty-six for men]. But now that we are married, his parents are unhappy that I am not yet pregnant. Can you give me some medicines?"

"I will give you herbs to strengthen your Qi, but you must be patient. Be happy with your husband and with your life. You will become pregnant soon enough. Do not be anxious."

Dr. Weng recognized that what was necessary here was reassurance, not necessarily medical intervention. But since this woman came with the expectation of receiving a prescription for a problem she perceived as an imbalance of Qi, Weng complied.

Family pressures to have a child can be considerable. However, now that the Chinese government insists that each family limit the number of its children to one, a new set of problems has arisen.

A thirty-year-old woman came into our acupuncture clinic to be treated for backache and fatigue. She was a thin, nervous, round-shouldered lady. Her gray, pleated trousers were far too big for her, and her belt was wrapped twice around her tiny waist. Her body was frail, and her hands were rough and calloused from physical labor. She looked tired and depressed.

"Good afternoon, Comrade Liu," said Dr. Zhang. "How are you today?"

"Fine, Dr. Zhang." Doctor and patient had obviously met before.

"Tell me, do you have any problems other than your backache and neurasthenia?"

"No," said Comrade Liu. Zhang began inserting acupuncture needles along the woman's back, neck, and arms.

Once again I broke the cardinal rule and began asking personal questions.

"Comrade Liu, would you mind telling me a little about your family?"

"Well, I have three children. Yes, three. I suppose you could say that is a problem, yes?"

"Why?"

"You see, my first child was a girl. My husband and I wanted a son. We had a second child. That was before the government limited the number of children we could have. Our second child was also a girl. That made two girls, and the government had set the limit at two children per family. But my husband and I and his parents and my parents, we all wanted a son to carry on the family name. So we had a third child. But it, too, was a girl. The fates have laughed at me. Now we have three girls, but ration coupons for only two. So buying rice, cotton, and some other goods we need . . . well, we cannot get everything we need, because we cannot receive the monthly bonus for families with the correct number of children. We barely have enough money. But worst of all," she looked at me plaintively, "sometimes the heart pains to be without a son."

As of 1980 the correct number of children for each family was lowered from two to one. This policy is said to be in the best interests of the nation, as China must control its population in order to survive. But customs die hard, and many couples would like to have more children.

Young adults in China are expected to abstain from sexual activity until they are married. Though authorities claim that premarital sex is nonexistent, it does go on and pregnancies among unmarried women do occur. It is important to note, though, that this problem is minuscule when compared with the problem of teenage pregnancies in the West.

At the Dong Zhi Men Hospital over the course of two weeks, a total of seven unmarried women received abortions. Six of the seven women were in their early twenties, had fiancés, and planned to get married as soon as they and their intended husbands reached legal age. These six women were escorted to the hospital by their husbands-to-be.

The doctors in the abortion clinic told me that, in circumstances like these, abortions would be performed in total confidence and that the women would be spared any public humiliation.

The seventh case, however, involved a young woman who had several boyfriends. She was known to have a bad reputation and was labeled a tramp. I was told that the work unit where she was employed would be informed of the woman's pregnancy and that she would be subject to the full force of public humiliation and disgrace.

"The Chinese people before liberation," said my instructor, "suffered greatly as a result of loose morals, prostitution, and venereal disease. We have conquered those enemies and will never permit them to return to China."

There are other examples of societal pressures unique to

modern China. For instance, although divorce is legal, it is highly discouraged. The family, the community, and the legal system make every effort to keep couples together. Those who insist on a divorce must contend with a society wholly unsympathetic to their actions.

People in China cannot move to other cities at will. A farmer who wishes to live in the city cannot simply relocate there from the countryside. All travel is restricted, geographic quotas are maintained, and people remain where they grew up unless they are "reassigned according to need." The millions of Chinese who were "reassigned" during the Cultural Revolution suffered a great deal of psychological stress.

A Chinese surgeon described his situation in the following letter to me:

"In your former lecture, you put forward some questions about social pressures in China and how these get resolved. Though my English is not good, I'll try to write something of my job and family as related to the pressure of separation.

"I graduated from medical school in 1965. I was sent to work in the countryside even though my parents and fiancée were in Beijing. I was not married yet, so I had to accept this situation. It was only after some time that I gradually got accustomed to being reassigned. I worked hard in the rural hospital and learned something new every day. There were patients to be taken care of, and besides work in the hospital I had to spend part of my time studying. I wrote frequently to my parents and my fiancée. That reminded me of my home and made me homesick.

"I got married two years after going to the countryside. As you know, families who are separated enjoy a vacation of twelve days a year. During that vacation I tried to stay home as long as possible. But the moment of parting was painful, especially for my wife.

"Some years later, I was sent to work in yet another country-side hospital. This was a larger hospital, but the work was even more tiring and the wages were the same. I remember my confused situation. I did not know what to do, so I consulted my friends. They said you must go to this new hospital; you must accept your new post. So, you see, I am a person who is easy to adapt himself to change.

"It was only after 1972, when my professional obligation was finished, that I yearned to return to Beijing forever. I felt home-sick, and the feeling grew stronger than ever. I talked to the director of my hospital and wrote reports asking to be reassigned to Beijing. The leader of my hospital sympathized with my separation from family. He approved of my leaving, but it was not to come about for another six years. It was indeed difficult to change my position, but I ended up a lucky fellow. There are still people in the countryside looking forward to returning home. As to how my problem was resolved in detail, I cannot tell you.

"Everyone has problems from time to time. Once old problems are resolved, new ones appear. I have been reunited with my family after thirteen years. Now I worry about new problems like my wife's professional difficulties. She works in a distant suburb and must use two hours to get to her working place. I think the saying 'There is no limit to one's wanting' may be correct."

What can China do for the patient with emotional pain or psychiatric disturbance? Some patients will neither discuss their problem nor seek medical attention. Some fraction of these patients will somatize their problem and seek treatment in the clinics of traditional or Western-style doctors. Others will consult with their immediate family, with their intimate friends, and possibly with trusted elders. A physician, however, is generally not one of the patient's principal confidants. The Chinese have used this support network of family, friends, and elders for thousands of years. Today in Communist China there is another member of the support team—namely, the political leader.

Every one of China's billion citizens belongs to some "unit" —either a commune or a factory or the like. Each unit has a complex hierarchy of political authorities. The political leaders are ultimately responsible for decisions about hiring, relocating, setting job quotas, and the like. These are the people with the power to change life circumstances for individual citizens. They can arrange for a change of jobs or a change of supervisor. Doctors do not have this authority. My surgeon friend from the Beijing Second Medical College made this point well:

"What can be done with patients who suffer from anxiety or depression? Conditions are so very different in China and America. In China a man or a woman who might have some problem to resolve would first consult with his family and friends and then ask a responsible political leader to help him with the problem. Whether the problem has to do with job or family does not matter. In either case the patient would not consult with a doctor, as a doctor does not and cannot resolve these problems in China. Personal problems might make people depressed, but the doctor is limited to administering medicines. Most problems that have something to do with anxiety or depression are best resolved by family or by political leaders—not by doctors."

Visiting a Psychiatric Hospital

Patients at risk of doing harm to others or to themselves (e.g., frankly psychotic individuals, schizophrenics, and suicidal patients) are hospitalized in psychiatric institutions. In Beijing I visited the An Ding Psychiatric Hospital, a facility that accommodated two thousand psychiatric inpatients.

The first ward housed sixty chronic patients dressed in black-and-white striped hospital pajamas, seated on their small cots, reading comic books, playing cards, or staring off into space. A heavy young woman in the back of the room was jumping up and down on her bed, waving to me. I walked over to say hello. Her hair was disheveled, her shoes were on the wrong feet, and she had difficulty focusing her eyes. She stopped bouncing long enough to reach out and give me a powerful handshake. She said she wasn't sick, had been stricken with schizophrenia before but had cured herself, and would be going home very soon and would never be sick again. She asked me what I thought. Before I could answer, she went right on to another thought.

"I am from Beijing. Where are you from?"

"America."

This single word unleashed a flood of energy in her. "Long live American-Chinese friendship!" she shouted. "And the greatness of our two nations. Let us remember the historic meeting of our beloved Zhou Enlai and your President Nixon! Long live the willingness of the Chinese people to become true friends with the American people." Then her eyes landed on my school pin: *Beijing Institute of Traditional Chinese Medicine.* "Did China give you that pin?"

"Yes."

Her face changed, her eyes stood still, her jaw came forward, and her nostrils flared. She started to bounce again and screamed, "What have you given to my country? What have you given my homeland? Speak! Speak!"

A large female attendant rushed over to restrain her. Someone asked me politely whether I was ready to move on to the next ward.

The An Ding Hospital cared for patients with major psychopa-

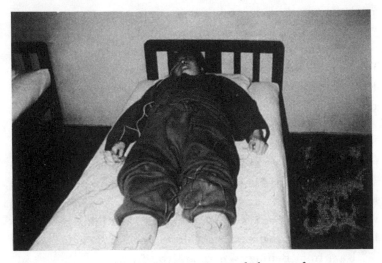

Electrical acupuncture—an experimental therapy for schizophrenia.

thology. I spent time with schizophrenics and manic-depressives in occupational- and recreational-therapy units.

With the exception of what we in the West would call insight-oriented psychotherapy (all those therapies whose essential method is discussion between doctor and patient), these patients received the same form of intervention used in the West. The An Ding psychiatrists prescribed drugs like lithium and Thorazine. They used electroconvulsive shock therapy and environmental therapy. They also employed traditional herbal remedies and electroacupuncture experimentally for all types of major psychopathology.

Following my tour of the psychiatric wards, I met Dr. Wu Zheng-yi, director of the hospital. Dr. Wu, an immaculately dressed, distinguished-looking man with silver hair, met me in the conference room next to his office. We sat on large, art

192

deco gray sofas and sipped jasmine tea.

Dr. Wu introduced himself in perfect English with an unmistakably American inflection. He had acquired his American accent during psychiatric training at the University of California at Berkeley in the 1940s. Since then he had been a practicing psychiatrist in Beijing. Dr. Wu's extensive training was rare among physicians in China.

The following are excerpts from my question-and-answer session with Dr. Wu Zheng-yi:

Eisenberg—Most of the articles I have read dealing with psychiatry in China were written during the Gang of Four period. They spoke of intense physical labor, regimented political therapy sessions, and psychiatric rehabilitation through the study of the late Chairman Mao's writings.

Dr. Wu—That era is over. The current trend includes the study of Western psychoactive drugs, occupational therapy, individual and group therapy, neurochemistry, neurophysiology, hereditary factors, as well as community and preventive psychiatry.

Q.—What is the main focus of your research?

A.—We are trying to determine the efficacy of our traditional medicines in the treatment of mental illness. We are evaluating the use of acupuncture and herbal formulas.

Q.—Do you have any preliminary findings?

A.—Our findings suggest that acupuncture is effective in the management of patients suffering from hallucinations, mania, and insomnia. But these findings are preliminary and the mechanisms remain unknown.

Q.—Why aren't you concentrating more heavily on the use of Western methods?

A.—We do use many Western methods, especially the newer psychotropic drugs. But you must remember that Western medicine was introduced to China only eighty years ago, while traditional methods have been used for treating mental illness for thousands of years. Part of our task must be to clarify and study the many valuable old methods of traditional medicine in our country.

Q.—What methods, if any, do you employ as a matter of course here?

A.—As you noticed, schizophrenics and manic-depressives receive the same drugs that you use in Western psychiatric hospitals. A few cases of severe depression are treated with insulin shock or electric shock therapy.

Q.—What are the comparative rates of mental illness in China and in the West?

A.—There are no published statistics, but I believe our frequency of schizophrenia is similar to yours. The rates of suicide, depression, alcoholism, and senile dementia are somewhat lower here than they are in the West. This is only my personal observation, and I am not certain why there is this difference in the rates of mental illness between the two populations.

Q.—Are there many psychiatric problems related to sexual dysfunction in China?

A.—I have observed some. But these problems usually do not find their way to a psychiatrist. Patients who suffer from impotence, frigidity, or sexual anxiety, for example, usually seek the attention of a gynecologist, urologist, neurologist, or traditional Chinese doctor.

Q.—It is my understanding that Chinese patients prefer to view their problems in terms of somatic [bodily] dysfunction rather than in terms of psychiatric problems. Do you find this to be the case?

A.—Yes, Chinese patients do have a tendency to somatize.

Q.—Does this pose stumbling blocks for the psychiatrists in your country?

A.—Yes, but psychiatry has only recently been introduced in medical and postgraduate medical education. Doctors of traditional medicine do not generally understand the field of psychiatry, nor can they be expected to recognize those patients who might conceivably be helped by it. Certainly, this lack of exposure to formal psychiatric training results in failure to identify and refer mentally ill patients to psychiatrists. But, then, we don't necessarily agree with most Freudian theories, either. Traditional medicine has its own assertions and classifications of mental illness. Each theory regarding mental illness has its good and bad sides. We cannot accept everything you offer as the truth, and you, on your part, should not discount the valid means for treating mental illness that we may have to offer. Certain drugs rigorously tested and found effective in your country are also effective here. Lithium, for instance, in controlling manic-depressive illness. This is a tribute to the Western scientific method. We welcome your help in exploring a methodology of treatment suitable for our population. But we must not forget that the vast majority of psychiatric problems have no specific cures, just a multiplicity of therapeutic approaches. Not all of the approaches used by Western psychiatrists are applicable to the customs and beliefs of Chinese patients."

Chinese psychiatry shies away from insight-oriented psychotherapy. This reluctance stems in part from a cultural disinclination to discuss personal matters outside the family and from a cultural bias that defines mental illness in terms of an inner disharmony of Yin and Yang. Chinese psychiatric patients can comprehend their mental disorders far better in terms of excesses or deficiencies of Qi than in terms of oedipal complexes or Eriksonian developmental stages. Western psychotherapeutic approaches have not been widely implemented in China. If they are, they will very likely meet great resistance.

The following is an excerpt from a letter that an internist in one of my English classes wrote as an exercise: "Dear Dr. Ai: . . . Last week you talked about Freud and his theory of the unconscious. It was very interesting. . . . We went to the library, but we did not find any data. Freud is not here. . . ."

Fourth Encounter: Testing Qi

From 1980 to 1983 I was in America doing an internship and residency in internal medicine. During this time two seemingly unrelated medical trends were emerging at opposite ends of the world. In China the trend involved Qi Gong; in the United States, behavioral medicine. Both sought answers to the question of how psychological attitudes affect the natural course of human illness. That these two trends were intimately related and evolving simultaneously went unreported in the *New England Journal of Medicine*. But related they were and continue to be.

I returned to China in July 1983 at the invitation of one of my former teachers, Dr. Herbert Benson, director of the Division of Behavioral Medicine at Harvard Medical School. Dr. Benson is a pioneer in the field of behavioral medicine, a seasoned researcher in the influence of mental activities on physiology. He was trained as a cardiologist and in the 1960s began his studies on the physiological effects of meditation. His research led him to the discovery of a physiological pattern that he termed the relaxation response. He first detected it in the lower pulse and blood pressure and the reduced oxygen demand of those practicing transcendental meditation. With further investigation Benson proved that this physiological response could be obtained by anyone who followed four basic steps. These simple steps, traced to the religious practices of many organized religions, including those of Jews, Christians, Muslims, and Hindus, had profound health-promoting effects. The steps are (1) sitting quietly, (2) concentrating on one's breathing, (3) repeating a word, thought, or idea, and (4) passively disregarding other thoughts as they come to mind and returning to the initial repetitive word, thought, or idea.

Behavioral medicine brings science to bear on an age-old question—How do our life-style and our thoughts affect our health? Benson's work marked a breakthrough because he used the relaxation response successfully in the management of hypertension. He next studied monks from India and Tibet, documenting physiological changes that came about as a result of the relaxation response. But Benson knew little about traditional Chinese medicine and was keen to investigate the area of Qi Gong.

After returning from China in 1980, I shared my observations with Dr. Benson. He was interested but skeptical. He thought my accounts accurate, but he remained fearful that my observations had been altered by my enthusiasm. Benson's interest in Qi Gong was twofold. He wanted to know, first, whether this age-old practice was based on the relaxation response and/or other health-promoting reflexes and, second, whether practitioners of Qi Gong were capable of altering their physiology in ways that Western medicine had not yet encountered. Benson and I drafted a letter to Director Lin Hai of the Shanghai Qi Gong research unit, the place where I had witnessed a demonstration of psychokinesis. We suggested collaborative studies and an exchange of personnel. For unclear reasons we never received a reply.

A year later Benson proposed a formal medical expedition to China, specifically to investigate Qi Gong therapy. To the amazement of everyone involved in the project, the Chinese authorities accepted this proposal. Our hosts would be the Chinese Ministry of Health and the Beijing Institute of Traditional Chinese Medicine—my alma mater. Only three years earlier Qi Gong had been a state secret.

On the plane ride to Hong Kong, I thought about the inexplicable observations I had made in 1979–1980: the Qi Gong master in Beijing who moved the lamp without touching it; the Qi Gong master in the Shanghai research unit who moved a dart without touching it; the clairvoyance of the Wang sisters; the reports of Qi Gong masters who emit energy at will and use it for therapeutic purposes.

At the Beijing Institute of Traditional Chinese Medicine, clinicians and scholars had attempted to convince me that Qi, the principle of vital energy at the core of Chinese medical theory and practice, had a physical reality that Western science would inevitably recognize. Back in the United States this concept seemed more *Star Wars* fantasy than fact.

We arrived in Shanghai, where we spent two days. The first day we visited the Qi Gong Hypertension Unit of the Rei Jin Hospital. The hospital was built in the early part of this century by European missionaries. The walls sloped; the ceilings showed their age. In this dilapidated hospital, Qi Gong research had been under way continually since 1958. Several thousand patients with hypertension had been instructed in the basic exercises of Qi Gong. According to Dr. Wong Chong-xing, director of the research team, the majority of the hypertensive patients enjoyed a dramatic improvement of their blood pressure control. A series of studies involving 1,800 patients suggested that the daily practice of Qi Gong lowered blood pressure, pulse rates, metabolic rates, and oxygen demand. They indicated, too, that levels of dopamine β-hydroxylase (an enzyme controlling neurological activity) were significantly reduced in practitioners of Qi Gong.* The Qi Gong exercises consisted of specific physical movements that resembled those of Tai Ji Quan, and also involved relaxation and meditation techniques and meticulous attention to abdominal breathing. Patients with high blood pressure learned these exercises over a span of two weeks, then returned to the hospital periodically for follow-up training and observation.

The physiological studies done on Qi Gong practitioners in Shanghai were nearly identical to the investigation of the relaxation response that Benson carried out in Boston years later. The odd thing was that neither group had known of the other's existence. Benson was struck by the uncanny similarities. He was convinced that the relaxation response was an essential aspect of Qi Gong exercise and wanted to learn of its clinical implementation in China.

In the 1950s and 1960s Qi Gong had been taught not just in the Rei Jin Hospital but also in dozens of other hospitals throughout Shanghai. Its use was not restricted to the treatment of hypertensive patients. Qi Gong had been applied to patients with asthma, peptic ulcer disease, neurological disorders, arthri-

---

* Personal correspondence, Dr. Wong Chong-xing, Shanghai Hypertension Research Unit, July 1983.

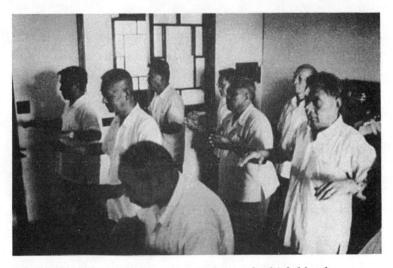

Internal Qi Gong exercises as a treatment for high blood pressure.

tis, gastrointestinal illness, and even fatal cancers. "What were your results?" asked Benson. Dr. Wong was vague in his response. He urged us to wait until our meeting with our Beijing hosts to discuss the matter in greater detail.

We asked the doctors in Shanghai what they knew about the concept of "external Qi," that is, the emission of Qi at will by a practitioner of Qi Gong. The Rei Jin physicians believed that this phenomenon was real. "External Qi is merely what we call consciously directed Qi. It is an extension of one's internal Qi, and we have all experienced sensations of directing Qi to particular parts of our bodies." The scientists in the Rei Jin Hospital had made preliminary measurements of infrared radiation projected from various portions of the body of Qi Gong practitioners. They had also documented increases in body surface temperature at the identical anatomical sites. It was impossible to know whether the infrared radiation represented a true emission of energy or merely a manifestation of the increase in body surface temperature. This kind of research, we were told, was going on elsewhere, but we were given no details.

The next morning, we visited the Shanghai First Medical College to talk with members of the Department of Acupuncture Research. The group was composed of physiologists and biochemists. These scientists had begun their research twenty-five years earlier with physiological investigations of acupuncture analgesia. We asked them whether they believed in the existence of Qi as a physical reality and in the ability of Qi Gong experts to emit energy at will. "We are physiologists trained in physiology, so we do not believe in the emission of external Qi. It makes no sense to us on the basis of Western medical science." These physiologists shared the biases of their American counterparts.

Later that same day, at the Eye, Ear, Nose, and Throat Hospital of the Shanghai First Medical College, our delegation got a glimpse of the unexplainable side of Qi Gong. The meeting took place at the invitation of Dr. Guo and Dr. Ni, two ear, nose, and throat specialists trained in China and the United States. These doctors were no strangers to the scientific method.

After tea and preliminary speeches, Dr. Guo and Dr. Ni reviewed a study they had performed on a Qi Gong healer said to be capable of emitting external Qi for therapeutic purposes. The experiment involved children with severe myopia (nearsightedness). Eighty myopic children ranging in age from twelve to fifteen were selected at random from the ophthalmology clinic. Each child underwent a thorough eye examination, including a precise measurement of vision, anterior chamber dimension, and corneal curvature. The natural course of this condition, myopia, when studied in children suggests that vision typically stays the same or gets worse and rarely improves spontaneously. This is because nearsightedness has to do with a defect in the curvature of the eye itself. The eighty children selected for this study were divided into four groups. The first group received no treatment. The second received placebo eye drops. The third was instructed in the practice of Qi Gong, the exercises being similar to those used for adult hypertensive patients; the children in this group attended classes for two weeks. The fourth group was treated by the Qi Gong master, who spent twenty minutes a day with one hand in front and one hand behind each child's head "emitting external Qi" in the direction of the eyeballs.

Dr. Guo and Dr. Ni proceeded to cite the findings of the study. Of the nontreated and placebo groups, none of the forty children had improvement of vision after two months. Of the twenty children who were taught Qi Gong exercises, two showed improvement in vision on the basis of multiple visual criteria. The research group speculated that so few had improved because the children were too young to concentrate on the meditative aspects of Qi Gong. Of the twenty nearsighted children treated by the Qi Gong master using external Qi, an astounding sixteen showed marked improvement in vision. This was again confirmed by multiple visual criteria. The ear, eye, nose, and throat staff admitted they were baffled by these preliminary results.

The next order of business was a demonstration by one of the school's Qi Gong masters, a Dr. Zhou. Like the other Qi Gong masters I had met, Zhou had a striking physical presence. He was a muscular man with a prominent neck and massive forearms. His face was calm, his eyes piercing, and his demeanor self-assured.

Zhou demonstrated his external Qi Gong on a young woman. She was a frail, giggling teenager wearing a summer dress and plastic shoes. It was unclear how this woman had come to meet Zhou or how many times she had been "treated" by him previously. We were told that the woman was "highly responsive" to

Zhou's external Qi and had for this reason been selected for the demonstration.

The girl stood in the middle of the conference room with hands at her sides, eyes closed, and feet together. She relaxed in silence. For several seconds she stood there doing nothing while Zhou walked around her in a circle, studying the girl's body as if it were a rare sculpture. Then Zhou brought his massive right arm up to about seventy-five degrees, his palm extended and fingers pointing at the girl. Her body began to move. She took short, spasmodic steps first forward, then right, then left; each time she had minimal losses in balance. She appeared to be in a trance, but whether it was feigned or induced none of us could tell. Over the next few minutes her movements were progressively less inhibited. She lunged forward and back, nearly falling. As each part of her body moved, Zhou's fingers and eyes made a parallel motion. Because these movements were so perfectly synchronized, it was impossible to say who was directing whom. After five minutes of lunging and tripping and twisting, Zhou took his hand and placed it on the young girl's neck to "release the excessive buildup of energy caused by the exercise" and, thus, ended the demonstration. The girl awoke and spoke of feeling totally relaxed but absolutely controlled by physical forces emanating from Zhou. The demonstration seemed an absurd hoax. I began to think we were witnessing a great sham.

The demonstration was repeated on a young man, who spun, pirouetted, and lunged about like a marionette, as the girl had done. After this demonstration, I interrupted the master and asked a question.

"Excuse me, Dr. Zhou, perhaps before you are too tired, you would agree to direct your external energy at one of us—at Dr. Benson, for example. Would this be possible?"

"Yes, I could do this," said Zhou without hesitating.

"All right," said Benson, removing his glasses and preparing himself for the highlight demonstration of the day. "Let's see how this works."

Benson stood in the middle of the large room, hands at his side, head slightly bowed, and feet together. Benson remained motionless, closed his eyes, and performed his own relaxation exercise. Zhou approached him cautiously, then aimed his arm at the Harvard professor's midsection. Benson appeared very relaxed, almost in a trance. Then he began to move. He swayed a bit from side to side, lost his footing, and tripped. He did not fall, but was clearly off balance. Zhou's arm tracked Benson's every movement, just as it had tracked those of the young girl and the young boy. Once again, it was impossible to know who was leading whom. Benson then began to twist his hips, first to the right, then to the left. He swiveled 180 degrees with awkward jerks. Benson smiled an uninterpretable smile. Zhou smiled in response, but Benson, whose eyes were closed, could not see this. After five minutes of bizarre motion, Zhou stopped the exercise, placed his right hand on Benson's neck, massaged it, and performed what he called a "removal of excess of Qi." Benson opened his eyes, shook his head, and sat down to address the audience. He described the peculiar sensations he had had during the demonstration. One was that of physical pressure seemingly coming from Zhou. In response to this pressure, Benson had voluntarily moved in an effort to resist Zhou's actions and test Zhou's strength. Benson said that he had initiated all of his own movements and was not convinced that Zhou could move him in any direction against his own will. On the other hand, the fact that Benson had any sensation of pressure from Zhou was interesting.

In the end the demonstration did little to shake Benson's

profound skepticism of man's ability to emit external energy. "It was all too subjective," said Benson. "Judgments cannot be made on the basis of subjective feelings alone. What we need is objective, reproducible data."

I had wanted to return to the Shanghai Institute of Traditional Chinese Medicine. It was there that I had three years earlier seen a demonstration of psychokinesis. This demonstration, performed under the direction of Dr. Lin Hai, a prominent Chinese scientist, was still etched in my mind. Benson and the rest of our delegation also wanted to visit Lin's Qi Gong research unit. Unfortunately, such a meeting had not been prearranged, and our hosts apologized for being unable to schedule it on short notice. Underneath the polite apologies, I scented the elusive odor of Chinese politics. Our Shanghai hosts reminded us that we were official guests of the *Beijing*, not the *Shanghai*, Institute of Traditional Chinese Medicine. The two "units" had limited contact. If we were patient, we would certainly see examples of external Qi Gong in Beijing.

The suspense of waiting raised doubts whether we would learn anything of value from this eccentric expedition to China. We were helpless before the subtleties of Chinese politics. And politicians, not Qi Gong researchers, were ultimately responsible for what we would see.

At the Beijing airport, representatives of the Beijing Institute of Traditional Medicine, the All-China Institute of Traditional Chinese Medicine, and the Beijing Qi Gong Society and the director of foreign affairs of the Chinese Ministry of Health gave us a warm welcome. A tentative schedule of meetings featured several demonstrations of internal and external Qi Gong. Things seemed to be looking up.

We checked into the Beijing Hotel and over dinner engaged

in our favorite pastime—speculation. We speculated as to whether Qi Gong represented more than the relaxation response, whether there was truth to the concept of "vital energy" within the body, and whether it could be regulated to alter the natural course of illness. We wondered what experiments could convince us that external Qi was a reality. Why the Chinese had agreed to our visit in the first place remained a mystery.

The next morning at six, we arrived at a local Beijing park for demonstrations of Qi Gong exercises. We noticed that our group was being videotaped for Chinese television. Five Qi Gong masters, powerful men with crushing grips, welcomed us at the park entrance. The water on the lake was calm as glass, a slate-gray backdrop for bright-red water lilies. Evergreen trees lined the banks. Scattered through the park in groups of fifty or a hundred were several thousand people. Some stood motionless, with eyes closed, breathing in precise patterns. Others performed Tai Ji Quan–like movements under the direction of Qi Gong instructors. These were the Qi Gong converts—thousands of avid practitioners studying Qi Gong at dawn. Most of them, we were informed, were cancer patients. What were thousands of terminally ill people doing studying Qi Gong at 6:00 A.M.? They were taking part in a popular revolution that had recently swept the Chinese nation.

The magnitude of the popular Qi Gong movement was staggering. In Beijing alone, more than 1.3 million people practiced one form of Qi Gong exercise daily. Other schools of Qi Gong had their own daily adherents. National figures had not been tabulated, but estimates of the number of Qi Gong practitioners ranged into the tens of millions.

Every morning at dawn, these millions of Chinese practice a three-thousand-year-old exercise that combines the motions of

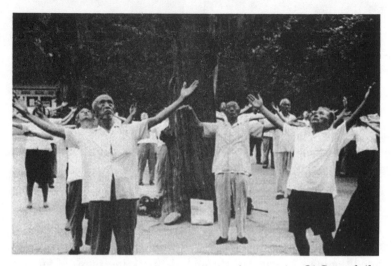

Some of the millions of cancer patients who practice Qi Gong daily.

Tai Ji Quan with meditation, relaxation, careful attention to breathing, and a specialized series of exercises that enable the practitioner to direct his or her internal energy throughout the body. In modern Western terms, Qi Gong combines aerobic conditioning, isometrics, isotonics, meditation, and relaxation. Chinese insist that by practicing Qi Gong one can significantly alter the natural course of illness.

A key figure in the Qi Gong popular movement is an eighty-year-old former cancer patient, Madame Guo. She claims to have had a gynecological malignancy when she was in her thirties. On the advice of gynecological experts in China and abroad, Madame Guo underwent several operations. Her pain, weight loss, and malaise persisted, and further surgeries were recommended. Madame Guo opted for a less conventional therapy and decided to study Qi Gong. Her cancer abated after a prolonged practice of Qi Gong.

Guo's conviction that Qi Gong had healed her terminal illness motivated her to teach the techniques to others. Her work began in earnest around 1970. Since then, Guo has taught Qi Gong to many thousands of enthusiastic patients, all of them reportedly suffering from terminal disease and the psychological devastation that accompanies these diagnoses. Seven days a week Guo leads Qi Gong classes. Her fame as a healer has swelled class size to the hundreds. A short, stocky, coarse-voiced lady, Guo wore a brightly patterned blue dress, the Chinese equivalent of a muumuu, when we met her. She was convinced Qi Gong could change the course of illness for many terminally ill patients.

In the 1970s Guo performed her own makeshift clinical studies on the efficacy of Qi Gong. Her methodology was primitive from the standpoint of Western science. In her examples, she allowed people with various illnesses, including cancer, asthma, ulcers, and rheumatologic disease, to *choose* which therapy they wished to have. Patients selected either (a) Qi Gong alone, (b) Qi Gong and Chinese medicine, or (c) Qi Gong and Chinese medicine combined with Western medicine. Her study was flawed from a Western perspective because the selection of patients was highly biased by patients' preferences and belief systems. A superior study design would have included a randomized selection of patients. We discussed these points with Madame Guo, who acknowledged that her research skills were deficient. She said she would be delighted to work with us to redesign a clinical study that could prove or disprove her assertions about the efficacy of Qi Gong therapy. We agreed to discuss this with the Ministry of Health.

After leaving the park, we were taken to the Institute of Traditional Chinese Medicine, where a series of introductory lectures on the history of Qi Gong added a valuable perspective to our trip. The practice of Qi Gong is said to have originated

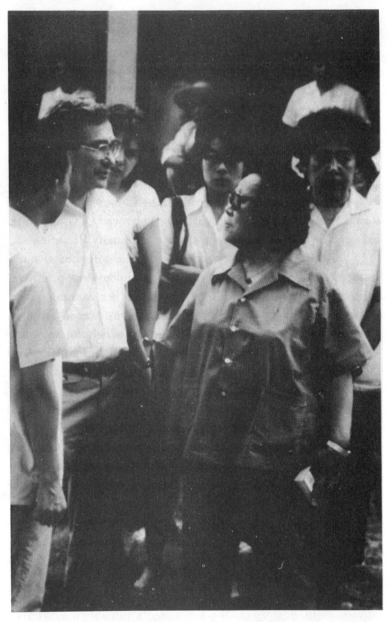

Dr. Herbert Benson with Madame Guo, a Qi Gong master famous
for treating cancer patients.

three thousand years ago. Its written history dates back to the period of the Warring States. It is mentioned in great detail in *The Yellow Emperor's Classic of Internal Medicine.* Chinese Daoists originated the technique, but Indian Buddhists influenced later Qi Gong practices.

All of China's famous scholars and philosophers, including Confucius, Lao Ze, and Mencius, were students of this technique.

Two kinds of Qi Gong practice were described. "Internal Qi Gong," was the manipulation of energy flow within one's own body by means of exercise. "External Qi Gong" meant the ability to project one's internal Qi toward another body. I had become familiar with these during my earlier visits.

The theory and practice of Qi Gong were applied to traditional Chinese medicine. Acupuncture meridians were interpreted as conduits for Qi. Organ systems and diseased states revealed balances and imbalances of Qi. Herbal medicine, massage, and moxibustion developed as therapeutic attempts to regulate Qi within the human body.

Qi Gong predates all other martial arts. Its highly stylized, circular, flowing, physical movements over the centuries spun off such familiar patterns as Tai Ji Quan, Kung Fu (Wu Shu), and Tai Kwan Do. After learning these physical movements, a student of Qi Gong must study patterned breathing. *Qi Gong* literally means "breathing skill", as the character for *Qi* means both "vital energy" and "breath." The breathing techniques of Qi Gong are complicated and varied. Its deep, rhythmic respiration involves the slow inhaling and exhaling of air by means of control from the diaphragm, chest wall, throat, tongue, and nasal passages. After mastering both the breathing and the physical movements, the student is taught to "focus" his or her Qi at a point in the center of the body. This point, located roughly two inches below the navel and deep within the pelvis, is named the *dan tian* (vital center). It is from this vital center that Qi is said to emanate to other parts of the body. With practice, students should sense the presence of Qi at this point in the form of localized warmth or heat. With further practice, they should learn to direct Qi to distant portions of the body. The whole process is said to require one to three months to learn.

Chinese researchers are now studying more than 100 distinct variations of Qi Gong. Down through the centuries, however, more than 3,600 schools of Qi Gong have existed. The ancient records of Qi Gong practice in religious literature are vast and have not been catalogued in their entirety.

Qi Gong's modern history dates back only to 1950. At that time many viewed claims of Qi Gong's efficacy in remedying disease as too fantastic to be believed. Qi Gong, such skeptics argued in the 1950s, was no more than "damaging superstition." However, Mao Ze-dong's call for the integration of traditional Chinese medicine and Western medicine prompted the first scientific investigation of Qi Gong.

In 1953 the first Qi Gong sanitorium, under the direction of a Dr. Lu Zhen, opened in the city of Beidaihe. Other major research units were founded in Beijing and Shanghai, including the Rei Jin Qi Gong Hypertension Unit. In each of these centers patients received instruction in Qi Gong exercises.

In 1959, at a national symposium, representatives from sixty-four Qi Gong research units reported on their preliminary findings. They said that Qi Gong had shown dramatic clinical efficacy in the management of patients with hypertension, peptic ulcer disease, asthma, diabetes, coronary artery disease, chronic kidney disease, tuberculosis, peripheral vascular disease, neurasthenia, arthritis, bowel problems, and a host of other chronic maladies. Initial physiological studies documented that

Qi Gong practice could decrease pulse rates, blood pressure, oxygen demand, metabolic rate, and lactate production.*

Qi Gong practice and clinical research came to an abrupt halt in 1964 with the beginning of the Cultural Revolution. Over the next fourteen years, little work was done in this area. Not until 1978 did the Qi Gong research units revive.

In 1980 Dr. Lin Ya-gu of the Shanghai Institute of Traditional Chinese Medicine published his initial work on the measurement of external Qi, in the *Shanghai Journal of Traditional Chinese Medicine.* †

In 1981 an internist working at the Beijing Institute of Traditional Chinese Medicine, Dr. Fong Li-da, published an article entitled "The Effects of External Qi on Bacterial Growth Patterns."‡ According to this study, a Qi Gong master capable of emitting external Qi was instructed to use his Qi to kill or promote the growth of bacteria. The experiment was rather simple in design. Three test tubes with equal numbers of *E. coli,* a common bacterium, were handed to the Qi Gong master. One tube was the control. After he held this tube, the Qi Gong master simply placed it on the laboratory bench, having done nothing to it. He then took one of two remaining tubes and attempted to "kill" all the bacteria in it by emitting "lethal Qi" for one minute. Finally, he grasped the third tube and for one minute subjected it to a "health-promoting" dose of external Qi. Over forty repetitions of the experiment allegedly showed that a "health-promoting" dose of Qi engendered a seven- to tenfold increase in the number of *E. coli.* A "lethal" dose of Qi lowered

---

* Valuable as these studies must be, the Chinese have never published them.
† Lin Ya-gu, "On the Thermovision of Ancient Chinese Traditional Training of 'Body Inner Force,' " *Shanghai Journal of Traditional Chinese Medicine,* March 1980, p. 38.
‡ In *China Qi Gong* magazine, 1 (1983): 36.

213

the number of bacteria by one-half or more. Dr. Fong, whom we met at the Beijing Institute of Traditional Chinese Medicine, presented these findings and was confident that they could be verified and reproduced in any laboratory.

In the past two years more work has been done on the measurements and characterization of what has been called external Qi. Within the Chinese Academy of Sciences physiologists, biophysicists, engineers, and high-energy physicists have taken part in investigating this phenomenon. Nuclear magnetic resonance scanners, CAT scanners, and other sophisticated electromagnetic devices have been employed to document and quantify external Qi Gong activity. Our hosts made available no details of this research. But they repeatedly asked Dr. Benson what electromagnetic machinery we would use if given the opportunity to research the nature of external Qi.

Qi Gong has become a mass phenomenon in the past five years. Qi Gong societies throughout the People's Republic maintain lengthy application lists of persons waiting to join Qi Gong classes in local districts. No epidemiological studies, however, have shown whether these millions of practitioners have changed their health status through daily Qi Gong exercise.

What to make of these reports and this popular explosion? The mere fact that more than ten million people get up at dawn to practice an ancient exercise does not prove that this practice can alter susceptibility to disease. The fact that the exercise is thousands of years old, and a hallmark of Daoist, Buddhist, and imperial Chinese scholarship, does not necessarily mean that human beings hold within them rivers, streams, and pools of "vital energy." There is also no objective proof that human beings can emit energy forces at will. Chinese reports of Buck Rogers–style experiments in which people kill bacteria, promote healing, emit particle beams, and display clairvoyance do not

214

prove that the phenomena truly exist. What we in our expedition group needed was a healthy dose of reproducible, objective data. We needed to see people directing their Qi at inanimate objects and altering those objects in the process. Subjective testimonials and reports of incredible experiments would not suffice.

The next morning at five-thirty we left the Beijing Hotel for the Temple of Heaven. Surrounding that temple is a park rich with pine and juniper trees. A shadowy clearing under rows of evergreens was the classroom for hundreds of Qi Gong faithful performing their daily routine. Five more Qi Gong instructors, all of them famous men, greeted us with powerful handshakes and grins of self-confidence. These were the most-skilled Qi Gong practitioners in Beijing. They had been looking forward to this meeting for months.

We sat down at an iron, patio-style table and were served lukewarm green lollipop-flavored soda in a bottle with a straw. This drink was the 5:30 A.M. eye-opener at official Qi Gong park visits. Liquid toothpaste would have been more palatable. Dr. Zhao Jin-xiang, founder and principal instructor of the crane school of Qi Gong—named for the movements of cranes and the largest in China, with millions of members—introduced us to his colleagues. Each morning the Qi Gong masters rotated through one of eighteen different Qi Gong practice centers throughout Beijing. At each center they lectured, demonstrated, and observed. Thousands of patients studied Qi Gong at the Temple of Heaven Park. Three had been asked to share testimonials of how Qi Gong had helped them. A patient said to have esophageal cancer spoke of his "cure" by Qi Gong. One suffering from bladder cancer told his story. A young woman with a chronic neurological infirmity explained that Qi Gong had allowed her to regain full neurological function after ten years of nearly total disability.

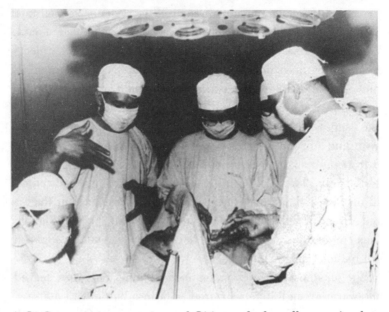

A Qi Gong master uses external Qi instead of needles to stimulate key acupuncture points for painless surgery. (Photo courtesy of Lin Ho-sheng, Shanghai Institute of Traditional Chinese Medicine)

We asked for a demonstration of external Qi. Would the Qi Gong masters mind "firing" at us? "We would be delighted," said Dr. Zhao Jin-xiang.

Dr. Benson's sixteen-year-old son, Gregory, and Dr. Margaret Caudill, an M.D.-Ph.D. working with Benson, volunteered to be the first subjects. Gregory and Margaret were told to stand side by side about six feet apart. Gregory was instructed to raise his right arm and Margaret her left, so that their fingertips almost touched and their palms were inches apart. One of the five Qi Gong masters, a former cancer patient himself, stood ten feet in front of them. He took several deep breaths, held them in, assumed a natural stance, and raised his right arm, aiming his

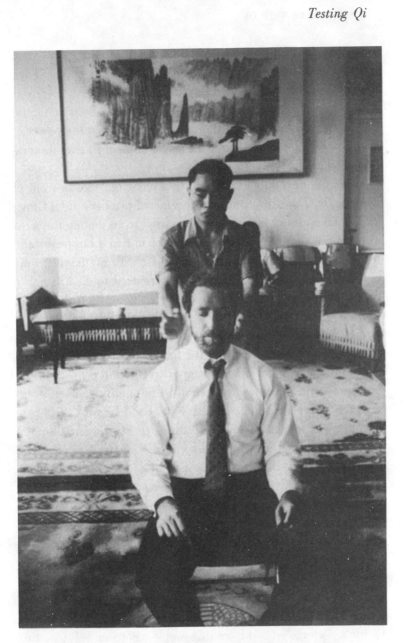

The author being "treated" with external Qi.

palm directly at the fingertips of Gregory and Margaret. Then he "fired" his Qi. Did they feel anything? Nothing at first. Then they noticed a numbness and tingling sensation. Next, there was a hint of pressure on their palms. Was this due to their maintaining an awkward position with arms raised? Was it the power of suggestion? Was it nothing at all? Was it a subjective observation, fool's gold?

I was the next subject. Sitting in a chair ten feet in front of me was Dr. Zhao Jin-xiang, the teacher of teachers of Qi Gong. Zhao's Qi-emitting powers were reported to be among the most awesome in China. A bear of a man, Zhao had a big frame and brawny arms and neck. I sat in the chair with my hands in my lap, closed my eyes, and attempted to relax. I told Zhao not to instruct me as to what I might feel. He agreed that this was a good idea and said, "Are you ready, Dr. Ai?" "I am ready," I replied. "Blast me, won't you? I don't want any half-felt sensations." As my eyes closed for the final time, I saw Zhao laugh behind a raised palm aimed in my direction.

For the first ten or twenty seconds, I felt nothing. Then it was my turn to get a dose of subjective poison. I began to feel pins and needles from my shoulders down to my fingernails. The sensations intensified, the pins and needles changed to electrical impulses. It was as if my hands had been plugged into a low-voltage socket. My fingers, wrists, arms, and shoulders tingled and grew numb. I said nothing, trying my damnedest to decide whether this was an illusory and transient sensation initiated by me or some atypical response to the energy being emitted by the popular hero sitting before me. "I feel something," I said to Dr. Zhao. "Give me everything you've got." In seconds the sensation of electrical impulses in my upper limbs grew in intensity. It was as though the voltage in the socket had been turned up to high. "Herb," I said, calling out to Benson, "I feel this

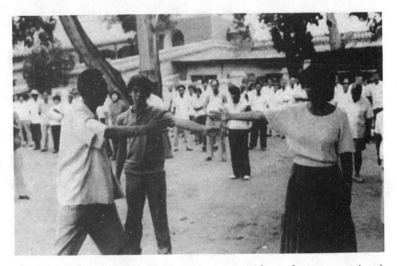

A Qi Gong master (and reported former esophageal-cancer patient) directing external Qi at Margaret Caudill, M.D., Ph.D., and Gregory Benson.

incredible sense of electricity shooting through my arms." Benson said nothing. Seconds later Zhao stopped, and the abnormal sensations ended abruptly. I was exhilarated but had no idea what to make of this demonstration.

Benson reminded me of the power of suggestion, which in my case is a confounding reality. As a medical student in one of Benson's classes, I had been assessed for my degree of hypnotizability. The general population falls into three categories: minimally hypotizable, moderately hypotizable, and extremely hypnotizable. I am extremely hypnotizable. Benson believed that this may have played a significant role in my feeling electrical sensations. He also speculated that my prior observations of Qi Gong activities, especially psychokinesis, and the feats of the Wang sisters may have been influenced by this hypnotizability. I could not argue this point and do not know what role, if any,

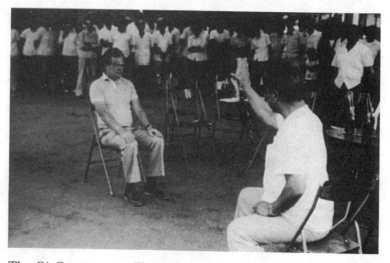

The Qi Gong master Zhao directing external Qi at Dr. Herbert Benson.

suggestibility played in my observations—all the more reason why objective data to prove or disprove the existence of Qi are critical.

Once again we reminded our Chinese hosts that we needed to see impartial demonstrations, ideally involving inanimate objects. This topic was a sensitive and delicate one to discuss, however, for we did not wish to give the impression that we were totally incredulous, nor did we want to be impolite.

Our hosts were clearly more fascinated with the use of internal and external Qi as modifiers of health than with discoveries of physical forces. They were trying to convince us that Qi Gong had the capacity to heal people, and they did not care how it did this. We wanted proof that their techniques were authentic. Our task would be much easier, we explained, if they could supply us with more objective data.

220

"Well, would you like to see me light a light bulb using my external Qi?" asked one of the Qi Gong masters. He was a former esophageal cancer patient.

"You mean to say that you can actually light a bulb just by emitting Qi?" I asked.

"Yes, anyone who has practiced external Qi Gong can do it. When you feel the Qi coming out of your arm, you can direct it at a bulb, and it always lights. Not any bulb, just fluorescent bulbs. Any fluorescent bulb will do. It's really not anything special. All of us can do it."

It is one thing to wake up at five-thirty in the morning on the other side of the world, to go to a park where thousands of cancer patients are practicing an ancient exercise, and to sip lukewarm soda pop while someone stands in front of you and gives you a sensation of mild electrocution. It is an order of magnitude more unsettling to be told that a fifty-year-old man has been cured of a lethal cancer (esophageal cancer is nearly 100 percent fatal) and that he has the ability to point his hand at a fluorescent fixture and light it up at will.

"Why not show us?" I said. "We'll be at the Beijing Institute of Traditional Chinese Medicine all afternoon. Why don't you meet us there and give us a demonstration?"

"Yes, okay, I'll be there," he said. If this odd fellow could do what he said he could, then I was certainly in the market for a new reality scale.

That afternoon Dr. Benson delivered his lecture on the relaxation response to the faculty of the Beijing Institute of Traditional Chinese Medicine. Benson first defined the physiology of the relaxation response. He then proposed that Qi Gong began with the relaxation response and that Qi Gong's therapeutic efficacy might be traced to this physiological mechanism.

During the informal discussions following the lecture, Benson told of his attempts to define the limits of our ability to use our minds to alter our bodily functions. Benson had studied practitioners of meditation, monks, and a variety of healers. He had wrestled with questions about the placebo effect and tried to measure physiological changes associated with healing. The Chinese had also been studying these phenomena but were not as forthcoming with their experiences. This no doubt reflected the political forces guiding and limiting our discussions.

As the afternoon session came to a close, we inquired about the whereabouts of the Qi Gong master we had met in the morning. We mentioned how important it was for us to see a demonstration of his light-bulb-lighting ability.

At precisely that moment our friend walked in the door smiling broadly, sweating, and panting, for he had just run from the nearest bus terminal. He had been on buses for more than two hours and had run all the way from the bus terminal for fear of missing us. I was delighted to see him, but our hosts did not appear terribly pleased. He was, after all, an unexpected and unfamiliar guest. Our hosts would need some time to review the matter before permitting this Qi Gong master to go ahead with any demonstration. They politely asked us to take a seat in the waiting room. We adjourned for some tea while our hosts disappeared down the corridors of the institute.

It was a crisis. Up to now the Chinese had been dealing all the cards. They had boasted quite a hand—including psychokinesis, health-modifying external energies, and clairvoyance. While they decided what to do, we sat by ourselves on doily-covered couches and sipped jasmine tea.

Could the Qi Gong master light a fluorescent bulb? What would it mean if he could? "Then, it's probably static electricity," said Benson. "You know, it's been shown if you generate enough static electricity, say, from rubbing your feet on the carpet, you can cause a flicker in a fluorescent bulb."

"Is that right?" I said.

"Yes, and that wouldn't require any new physics either."

Comrade Fang, our courteous interpreter, appeared in the doorway. "Excuse me for interrupting. I have good news for you. We will show you something very interesting now. Will you please come this way?"

They had actually decided to let us see this. "Herb," I said, "you know, I think they're going to show us the light." Herb smiled. His usually furrowed brow and serious mien changed. He took on a relaxed, puckish, mischievous expression. Enter Benson the hunter about to confront his favorite prey. His studies of mind-body interaction had kept him on the fringe paths of "healers" and "mystics" on several continents, in places far less hospitable than China. Armed with the scientific method and a healthy skepticism, Benson eagerly addressed this new claim. "Let's see what there is to see," said Benson calmly.

We walked down the green corridors to a one-bed dormitory room that belonged to the building superintendent. Makeshift drapes hugged the small window. The room was no bigger than a closet; a bed and a dresser monopolized most of the floor space. There were no carpets in the room or anywhere in the building. On the ceiling was a fluorescent fixture with no bulbs. On the bed was a five-foot, forty-watt fluorescent bulb. This bulb, we were told, had been taken from the fixture on the ceiling of the room. No other lights and no electronic objects were anywhere in sight.

Our Qi Gong friend was warming up next door in the office of the superintendent. With him was the vice-president of the Institute of Traditional Chinese Medicine, Dr. Gao He-ting, and the head of the Beijing Qi Gong society, Dr. Zhang Wan-you. We asked the Qi Gong master how this skill had been discovered. "Well, a few years ago, one of our Qi Gong teachers went to reach for a fluorescent bulb just after having completed his Qi Gong exercises, and the bulb lit up. Since then it has been fairly well known that anyone able to perform external Qi Gong can, with practice, project it at a light bulb and light it up. But we can do this only immediately after practicing Qi Gong. On some days it seems easier to light the bulb than on others. Oh, yes, for some reason we can't light bulbs if we're in a building and higher than the fifth floor. I haven't the faintest idea why this is so, but the fifth floor is as high as I or anyone I know can go and still light bulbs. Are you ready to see me light the bulb now?"

The room was only big enough for half of our group. Benson stood beside me in the corner of the room in front of the dresser and just behind the Qi Gong master. He walked into the room from the hall where he'd been exercising for about thirty minutes. His hands had a white powder on them. I don't know what kind it was. The Qi Gong master picked up the bulb with his left hand, gripped it about one foot from the left end, and held it in front of his chest. Bending his left elbow slightly, he held the bulb at about seventy-five degrees from the horizontal. "Close the door," he said. Benson kicked it shut. It was pitch black in the room, and we could see nothing, not even the outline of the Qi Gong master or the bulb. "Are you ready? I'm going to do it now," he said. "Yes," I said, "go ahead. We're all watching."

The Qi Gong master took three enormous breaths. The rush of exhaled air was the only sound we heard. We could see nothing. After thirty seconds of breathing, we heard a slap. The Qi Gong master's right palm slapped the bulb about one foot from the right end of the glass rod; then his palm hugged the bulb, traveling from right to left over about a foot of its length.

The sound of skin rubbing on glass could be heard as his hand rapidly traversed the midsection of the bulb. With the second or third slap, each of which took only a second, the bulb began to glow. The fluorescence followed a path from right to left directly in front of the Qi Gong master's hand as it traveled over the midsection of the bulb. The light followed the path of his hand precisely. Every time he slapped the bulb it fluoresced brightly. He repeated the motion five or six times in exactly the fashion described. Then he stopped and said breathlessly, "There, did you see it? Did you see it?"

We had seen it. Benson opened the door. The Qi Gong master was sweating profusely at this point. "I'm glad I could do it for you. I knew you didn't believe me this morning. I had to show you. I know that this seems very strange to you, but it is real and many people can do this."

Our Qi Gong friend went back to the superintendent's room to rest. He sat down on the couch, obviously exhausted, and asked for some water or tea. Dr. Gao He-ting, vice-president of the institute, appeared in the hallway and called to me. "Dr. Ai, you are the first foreign friends to see this demonstration. Amazing, isn't it?" "Yes, yes," I said. "Thank you very much for letting us share this with you. It is just the sort of demonstration we have wanted to see. Thank you again. We are most grateful."

It was late, the Qi Gong master was too exhausted to repeat his performance, and we were tired and had asked enough favors for one day. We said our good-byes for the evening and got on the minibus to return to the Beijing Hotel.

"What do you think, Herb?" I asked. "Well," he answered, "I think it's probably some form of static electricity. Or it's a fake. You know, we couldn't see anything in that room. Once the door was closed and it was black, a million and one things could have happened without our knowing it. You can't say anything about it. We had no control over any of this demonstration. If you tried to publish a description of this sort of observation in any scientific journal, critics would skin you alive, and they'd have a right to. I don't know what they just did. We'll have to talk to some physicists and magicians, and we'll have to see this done many times in a totally controlled environment before considering it anything new." Benson's armor remained unscathed.

The next afternoon we were to meet Vice-Minister Tan Yun-he of the Ministry of Health. We had been asked to present concrete proposals for future collaborative research on Qi Gong. Benson carefully reviewed what we'd seen and decided to propose two projects.

In the vice-minister's office Benson suggested that a collaborative U.S.-Chinese clinical study be designed and carried out in China with the guidance of American experts. There would be two parts to the proposed experiment: one testing the efficacy of Qi Gong in the treatment of hypertension, the other testing its efficacy in the treatment of documented lung cancer.

Benson also recommended that Qi Gong masters visit the United States to demonstrate their powers under controlled laboratory conditions. Vice-Minister Tan thought these were excellent proposals and delegated to Director Dong Yu-chang of the Bureau of Foreign Affairs the responsibility for their implementation. Subsequently, Director Dong said the Ministry of Health was interested in our collaborating on a documentary film introducing Qi Gong and the basics of Chinese medicine to the Western world. He told us that the sooner detailed negotiations could begin, the better. The Ministry of Health had scheduled a worldwide symposium on the science of Qi Gong in Beijing in 1985.

Making sense of these Qi Gong–related observations, assertions, and political invitations is no easy task. The concept of mind altering matter seems better suited to mythology or science fiction than to medicine or physics. And yet it is consistent with the Chinese principle that our thoughts influence our physical state profoundly.

There are several possible ways to explain the observations cited by Chinese authorities. First, one must dissect the practice of Qi Gong into its component parts. The principal form of Qi Gong is internal Qi Gong. This is the daily practice of age-old exercises easily learned and performed by anyone. Millions of Chinese now subscribe to this form of exercise for the preservation of health and the treatment of disease. Traditional Chinese medical authorities in the Ministry of Health believe that the daily practice of Qi Gong significantly alters one's susceptibility to disease and changes the morbidity or mortality associated with disease. Furthermore, these authorities are now asking Western medical researchers to help them prove their point through clinical studies. If they are wrong, then Western medical science will have lost nothing by participating in clinical studies. If they are correct, however, then it will be compelled to review its basic assumptions about the nature of health and illness.

If Qi Gong practice can be shown to decrease the prevalance or symptoms of disease and to increase survival time, the next question will be how Qi Gong accomplishes this. Is it the *belief* in the practice of Qi Gong, what we in the West would call the placebo effect, or is it the practice itself that directly alters health status? If it is the practice of Qi Gong directly, the next question will be which elements of this practice play a crucial role. A one-hour session of Qi Gong combines aerobic, isometric, and isotonic exercise with the relaxation response, meditation, guided imagery, and probably several unrecognized behavioral techniques. It evokes simultaneously almost every behavioral intervention known to Western medicine. Perhaps the synergistic effect of these techniques can alter human physiology (especially the body's immunoregulatory system) and thus influence the natural course of illness. If so, then Western medical practice may someday incorporate health-promoting techniques like Qi Gong therapy.

The other major component of Qi Gong practice is that of external Qi Gong. It is this aspect of Qi Gong that plays havoc with Western biophysical laws. The Chinese see external Qi simply as an extension of internal Qi. Internal Qi Gong supposedly enables a person to sense, regulate, and direct internal Qi within his or her own body. A small fraction of the practitioners of internal Qi Gong achieve a level of control of their internal Qi that enables them to emit this Qi externally. Not everyone who practices internal Qi Gong can ultimately learn to perform external Qi Gong. This achievement is not a predictable or well-understood phenomenon, according to Chinese medical experts.

Although the practice of external Qi Gong has a three-thousand-year history and although external Qi Gong practitioners have been mentioned in numerous Chinese medical texts, external Qi Gong was not investigated scientifically until 1978. The Chinese believe that in the past seven years they have proven the existence of Qi as a physical reality. They claim that it is evident in psychokinetic power, clairvoyance, and health-promoting energies. These assertions may spring in part from myth, self-deception, and heightened suggestibility. The Chinese want to believe in the existence of Qi. It has, after all, played a central role in their philosophy, science, literature, and art.

The suggestion that Chinese medical authorities would consciously dupe the Western scientific community is absurd. What could the Chinese Ministry of Health gain by presenting sham results and inviting American scientists to investigate them? If any one of the Chinese assertions is true, then China has taken a bold step toward illuminating new paths of understanding. Moreover, in inviting Western scientists to join their studies, Chinese authorities have expressed a commitment to international cooperation and friendship. They have displayed their willingness to have Qi Gong investigated and scrutinized according to the highest standards of modern scientific research.

It was only a decade ago that Chinese medical authorities introduced Western scientists to the practice of acupuncture. At first, acupuncture anesthesia was considered impossible. Next, acupuncture was labeled a placebo effect. Today we know that this placebo effect is based on a group of naturally occurring, morphine-like substances called endorphins and enkephalins. These brain substances appear to play a key role in modulating pain and other sensations. A whole new area of medical research has blossomed from such seeds as the first observations of acupuncture analgesia. Chinese Qi Gong could sow other seeds of great importance to the future of Western medicine. Negotiations are now under way for the testing of Qi Gong masters in American research laboratories.

The burden of proof remains on the Chinese. Research to date cannot prove or disprove Chinese claims about Qi Gong. Dr. Lu Bing-kuai, vice-president of the All-China Institute of Traditional Chinese Medicine and president of the Beijing Qi Gong society, told our delegation, "Qi Gong is an ancient practice, part of the 'national treasure-house' of traditional Chinese medicine. We have tried these past few years to understand it by means of modern scientific principles and techniques. We do not yet understand it and would like your help in defining the nature of Qi. It is my conviction that in order to fully comprehend Qi

Gong and those aspects of healing associated with Qi Gong, there must be more than the simple application of current scientific principles and methodology. What is necessary is a revolution in Western biomedical science."

We shall see.

The Marriage
of Chinese
and Western
Medicine

Thirty years ago Chairman Mao Ze-dong proposed that traditional Chinese and modern Western medicine join forces to improve the health care of the Chinese people. Such a union would be like a marriage arranged between rival kingdoms. To make the marriage, the two parties would have to overcome different languages, different philosophies, different practices, and generalized mistrust.

What broke off the engagement was the chaos of the Cultural Revolution. For nearly two decades the courtship remained in limbo. But over the past five years, the present Chinese government has begun to reconcile the squabbling parties.

It is not exactly a marriage made in heaven. Doctors running nuclear magnetic resonance scanning machines have little in common with doctors prescribing antelope-horn tea. Physicians from both schools have been guilty of condescension, defensive posturing, and ignorance of one another's methodology. There has been little mutual understanding and collaboration.

Doctors of Western medicine have no unequivocal proof that the practices of traditional medicine are clinically effective, nor do they know their potential side effects. For these reasons Western-style Chinese doctors do not use traditional Chinese medicine and do not refer patients to traditional practitioners. The opposite bias exists among traditional doctors, who understand little about Western medicine. This stalemate makes it impossible, in China as in the West, for doctors from either background to refer patients appropriately. Without detailed knowledge of which treatment, Chinese or Western, is most effective for specific diseases, patients will continue to receive less than optimal therapy. In order for the situation to change, the clinical efficacy of Chinese medical therapies must be scientifically confirmed.

The clinical research needed for such confirmation is a precious investment. It will clarify which techniques are most effective for which patients and enhance Western medicine's understanding of human physiology and health.

My clinical observations convinced me that acupuncture is effective in providing analgesia and controlling certain chronic-pain syndromes. We are beginning to understand the physiology of how acupuncture affects our central nervous system via endorphin/enkephalin pathways. If Chinese claims regarding the efficacy of acupuncture in treating non-pain-related diseases are correct, then acupuncture must have direct health-promoting effects on multiple-organ systems. This discovery will in turn lead to a new and improved understanding of the healing process.

Chinese massage is closely related to the practice of acupuncture. Acupuncture and massage make use of identical points on the body's surface, and both depend on predictable and precise connections between surface points and internal organs. The difference between these practices has to do with the type of stimulation each employs. If acupuncture can be shown to be clinically useful, it is likely that massage will also be proven effective. It would be particularly gratifying to show that massage is as effective as it is pleasant. Imagine how the doctor-patient relationship would improve if Western internists and pediatricians gave their patients a therapeutic massage along with a physical examination.

The majority of herbal preparations in China's vast pharmacopoeia have not yet been clinically evaluated with Western techniques. The testing of herbal remedies for their efficacy in managing common illnesses is a complicated task. But it can be done and will no doubt provide Western scientists with new pharmacologically active agents and an improved understanding of physiology.

The most intriguing Chinese therapy is that of Qi Gong. It is ancient, fundamental, and the most perplexing of Chinese therapeutic interventions. Various of its phenomena challenge the foundations of Western biomedical thought.

Qi Gong techniques epitomize the Chinese claim that the human psyche can influence susceptibility to disease and the natural course of illness. In the West we are beginning to investigate the relation between life stress and immunology, particularly as it pertains to cancer. Recent studies from the National Institutes of Health have shown that animals can be conditioned to regulate their immunodefenses (specifically their "natural killer" cell activity) in response to a given stimulus.* A good

---

* Dr. Novera Spector, research presentation at the First International Workshop on Neuroimmunomodulation, Washington, D.C., December 1984.

deal of research has focused on the relation between certain personality styles and particular diseases, for example, on that between Type A personality and heart disease. Western medicine has begun to ask whether and how meditation, biofeedback, the relaxation response, and faith alter human physiology. Researchers in behavioral science, psychosomatic medicine, endocrinology, and neurology are redefining the links between brain and body. This interdisciplinary field has been called psychoneuroimmunology. Three thousand years before the birth of the first psychoneuroimmunologist, Chinese doctors were struggling with the same mind-body relations.

Many technical problems complicate the testing of the clinical effects of traditional Chinese interventions. Subjective feelings of pain are still the principal means of assessing acupuncture. We have yet to improve objective markers, such as chemical changes or unequivocal alterations in physiology.

Herbal preparations are particularly hard to test. Chinese herbal therapies depend on diagnoses that have nothing in common with the diagnostic labels used in modern Western medicine. Recall that the "pneumococcal pneumonia" of the West may be "an excess of 'liver' fire" or "a deficiency of 'spleen' Yang" in China. Moreover, herbal prescriptions are changed from day to day as the patient's condition changes.

Qi Gong can theoretically be applied to all patients and all disease states. Clinical studies using hypertension and survival from cancer as objective end points may verify the claim that Qi Gong can reduce the susceptibility to disease as well as the morbidity or mortality associated with disease. If studies in American laboratories confirm any of China's assertions about Qi Gong masters' energy emission, psychokinesis, clairvoyance, or healing powers, we will need to adjust our sense of the limitations of the human body.

The marriage of Chinese and Western medicine offers Western scientists more than clinical techniques and physiological mechanisms, however. It also offers an alternative approach to health and illness.

Western medicine emphasizes intervention over prevention. Most Western research focuses on the intricacies of active disease; it gives comparatively little attention to the effect that life-style, personal disposition, and thoughts have on disease. China has taken a very different tack. In its traditional system, health is much more than the absence of observable pathology. Activity, diet, and psyche play critical roles in the Chinese perception of health and illness.

Technology and specialization have distanced doctors of Western medicine from their patients. Doctors are increasingly accused of being less sensitive; patients, of being less trusting. Traditional Chinese medicine offers valuable guidance in this area. It suggests that physicians present themselves as advisers and teachers of prevention rather than independent repair technicians. A Chinese physician's responsibilities classically involve more than the mere treatment of disease. They extend to prevention, teaching, emotional support, and recommendations about life-style. The Chinese patient—in theory, if not always in practice—is an active partner in the health care process. These ideals are not unknown in the West, but there they are not part of the daily attitude toward health care. If Western doctors and patients took nothing from China but a new vision of their relationship, they would owe a profound debt to traditional medicine.

The Chinese emphasis on life-style and psyche begs the question why people become ill when they do. Are we all merely sitting ducks waiting for the fatal combination of heredity, external factors, and the march of time to strike us down? Or are we primarily responsible for our own health because of the way we live and think? The answer probably lies somewhere between these extremes. The integration of Chinese and Western medicine should help improve our understanding of the cause and the course of human illness.

To study Chinese medicine is also to study the dynamics of the placebo effect. Many critics of traditional Chinese medicine feel that the efficacy of all Chinese therapy is based primarily on the power of the placebo effect. These critics insist that Chinese therapies work because patients believe they will work. The same statement applies to a host of Western medical practices as well. But instead of tracking down this phenomenon, instead of trying to understand exactly how a given patient's belief system alters his or her physiology, Western science has generally neglected the placebo effect. The term *placebo effect* is all too often used pejoratively to describe a clinical response that is poorly understood, unexpected, and unexplainable by means of existing theory.

Properly designed clinical studies of Chinese medical techniques would pinpoint which patients undergoing which therapies experienced the full-blown placebo effect. They would then examine these individuals for subtle physiological alterations. This research might prove invaluable to our understanding of the relation between attitude and disease.

The mind-body interaction also relates to our understanding of the concept of "healing." We must ask ourselves how healing takes place. In Western medicine a pill made of chemicals or biological substances has the power to heal. A surgeon's scalpel has the power to heal. Certain physical and mental exercises probably have the power to promote healing. The human body left to its own devices has the most remarkable healing powers of all.

The Marriage of Chinese and Western Medicine

What about other aspects of healing? Western scientists are beginning to acknowledge the placebo effect as a real, though poorly understood, mechanism of healing. What about unconditional faith, say, one's religious faith or one's faith in a particular doctor? Can this kind of unconditional faith also heal? Perhaps there are other dimensions to healing, ones that have nothing to do with pills, scalpels, exercises, or conscious beliefs. It is conceivable that human beings possess a capability to promote healing in one another. This kind of healing goes by many names: faith healing, shamanism, the laying on of hands, external Qi Gong. We don't understand these methods of healing. There is a science to be teased out of the debris of case reports and folk testimonials. Perhaps this kind of healing represents the ability of one person to alter the physiology of another without the assistance of drugs or scalpels. This kind of healing, which has always been an integral part of the doctor-patient relationship, remains an underexplored realm of modern medicine. To understand it will require the expertise of many fields, including medicine, psychology, physics, and philosophy. The art of healing is thousands of years old. The science of healing is still in the process of being born.

Although the incidence of specific diseases in China differs from that in the West, the patients are by and large the same —suffering from the same symptoms, the same diseased organs, the same tormented psyches. The Chinese and Western medical models are like two frames of reference in which identical phenomena are studied. Neither frame of reference provides an unobstructed view of health and illness. Each is incomplete and in need of refinement.

The differences between traditional Chinese and Western medicine have to do with the ways in which diseases are perceived, diagnosed, and treated. It remains to be seen how the two systems compare in terms of efficacy. But the systems need not be mutually exclusive. There is no reason why physicians cannot combine the finest elements of both schools. A Chinese proverb says, "The methods used by one man may be faulty; the methods used by two men will be better."

The current Chinese government has proposed that members of the Chinese and Western medical establishments come together to learn from one another and to work out the details of this marriage. On March 8, 1985, Dr. Wang Yu-ren, president of the Shanghai Institute of Traditional Medicine, signed a "Statement of Intention" proposing a series of collaborative U.S.-Chinese clinical trials. These trials will test the relative efficacy of Western medicine versus acupuncture, herbal therapy, and Qi Gong in the treatment of common illnesses, including malignant cancers. In addition, "the efficacy and mechanisms of Qi Gong as well as a physiological description of internal and external Qi will be evaluated clinically and from the standpoint of biophysics." Medical authorities in Beijing and Canton have since expressed their interest in identical studies.

This research, now in the planning stages, will occupy Chinese and Western scientists for many years. There are no guarantees, but the marriage of Chinese and Western medicine may bring both sides closer to their mutual goal of understanding health and eradicating those forces which lead to the deterioration of life.

Afterword

The ten years since this book was first published have seen an ever-rising flood of interest in traditional Chinese medicine and other forms of alternative medical care, from chiropractic and homeopathy to mega-vitamin regimens and a dizzying array of dietary supplements. The interest has arisen from the grass roots, as people across America and throughout the developed world have sought out alternative therapies and new models of healing and wellness.

Enlightened, fair-minded scrutiny of alternative medicine has continued to lag behind. Until very recently no one even knew how many Americans used alternative medical therapies in a given year, much less whether such therapies worked, or worked by virtue of more than the placebo effect. Fortunately, ignorance is giving way to real knowledge on such questions, and I am pleased to participate in the process.

About five years ago, with the support of the John E. Fetzer

Institute, several colleagues at Beth Israel Hospital in Boston and Harvard Medical School and I set out to document the extent to which Americans use alternative medicine on a regular basis. The results of our national survey, published two years ago in the *New England Journal of Medicine*, raised eyebrows in both the medical and the nonmedical community. For example:

- One in three respondents (34 percent) reported using at least one alternative therapy in the preceding year, and one-third of these saw providers of alternative therapy. Extrapolating from our survey, about 60 million adult Americans used at least one alternative therapy to treat a serious or bothersome medical problem in the year preceding our study.

- Seven out of ten people who used alternative therapies never told their medical doctors.

- The use of alternative therapy crossed all demographic groups we considered. There were no significant differences according to sex or insurance status, and only small variations according to the size of the community. The use of alternative therapy is more common among people 25 to 49 than those younger or older, less common among African Americans, and significantly more common among persons with some college education and annual incomes above $35,000.

- Among all the conditions studied, the frequency of use of alternative therapy was highest for back problems (36 percent), anxiety (28 percent), headaches (27 percent), chronic pain (26 percent), and cancer or tumors (24 percent, although use of alternative therapy for cancer and AIDS accounted for less than 3 percent of all use, consistent with their prevalence in the general population).

- Relaxation techniques, chiropractic, and massage were the alternative therapies used most often by the survey group.

240

· In 1990 Americans spent about $14 billion on alternative medical therapies—$10.5 billion paid out of pocket. This figure is comparable to the $12.8 billion spent out of pocket in 1990 for all hospitalizations in the United States.

· We estimated that over a twelve-month period, Americans made 425 million visits to offices of alternative medical practitioners (chiropractors, acupuncturists, homeopaths, etc.). This exceeded the number of visits made that same year to all internists, family practitioners, gynecologists, and pediatricians combined.

In sum we had quantified for the first time what Janis Claflin of the Fetzer Institute has called "an invisible mainstream" of U.S. health care, parallel to the conventional medical system.

A month after the *New England Journal of Medicine* publication, PBS aired the Emmy Award–winning documentary series *Healing and the Mind with Bill Moyers.* That series, also funded primarily by the Fetzer Institute, ushered in a second tidal wave of popular debate. Do alternative medical therapies work? Can the mind predictably alter the body in ways that change the course of health or illness? Given the country's response to *Healing and the Mind,* it was clear that tens of millions of Americans wanted to know more about alternative medicine.

I was delighted to serve as a principal adviser to the series, guiding Bill Moyers through the baffling labyrinth of traditional Chinese medicine. Often he and I visited the same practitioners you've met in the preceding chapters. No one could ask for a better companion in these travels than Bill Moyers. His keen interest balanced a healthy skepticism, and both flowed from his deep concern for others and his open-mindedness. I value the opportunity that *Healing and the Mind* provided to introduce Bill Moyers, and through him millions of Americans, to the intriguing possibilities in traditional Chinese medicine.

A few months after *Healing and the Mind* was first broadcast, Senator Tom Harkin, then chair of the Senate Health Appropriations Subcommittee, scheduled a hearing in Washington to discuss funding for alternative medicine research. At that time, Senator Harkin and several congressional colleagues heeded their constituents' concerns and asked that the U.S. National Institutes of Health evaluate alternative medical therapies. Towards this end, Congress wrote into law, and provided initial funding for, the Office of Alternative Medicine in the National Institutes of Health.

I was called to testify before Senator Harkin's subcommittee. I told the senators that we needed one or more centers, in the midst of our finest medical institutions, devoted to the rigorous and fair evaluation of alternative medical therapies. The creation of such centers would constitute an unprecedented collaboration involving some of the country's best clinical researchers working alongside practitioners of alternative medicine. With fair yet rigorous trials, these centers would neither condemn nor advocate alternative therapies, but would seek to understand whether and how these techniques work.

Doctors, nurses, and allied health professionals need this knowledge if we are to advise our patients effectively. There is nothing more frustrating than being unable to answer a patient's question: "Doc, so do you think this [alternative therapy] will help my problem?"

To paraphrase David Sackett, a respected professor of medicine, medical treatments can be recommended based on induction, deduction, or seduction. Induction flows from empirical observation. An herb or a vitamin or a particular diet seems to help a number of people with a particular problem and is therefore recommended on the basis of repeated observation. Deduction refers to a controlled experiment, as we've seen in earlier chapters—for example, where half the patients get the herb or drug or vitamin, and half receive a placebo. Deduction represents the "gold standard" of medical inquiry.

Seductive logic is responsible for much of alternative medicine's appeal. This is the world of anecdote. For example, if my mother's cousin's brother's college roommate suffered for years from incurable problem X; and if after a few minutes with an acupuncturist in New York or a massage therapist in Miami the problem disappeared, seductive logic tells us that this therapy did the trick. Anecdotes can and do provide the fuel for productive lines of inquiry. But they can also lead to disappointing dead ends.

As I wrote in the earlier chapters of this book, it will take the best scientific researchers to design studies to distinguish useful from useless interventions. The U.S. government has not yet funded a center devoted to the fair yet rigorous evaluation of commonly used alternative therapies. But my colleagues at Beth Israel Hospital and Harvard Medical School and I have taken up the challenge. On April 1, 1995, we formally inaugurated the Center for Alternative Medicine Research at Beth Israel Hospital, under the joint aegis of Beth Israel Hospital and Harvard Medical School.

The center will bring together leading scientific researchers and practitioners of alternative medicine to evaluate alternative therapies one by one. We'll try to understand which are safe, effective, and capable of cutting medical costs for individuals and for society as a whole. A new Beth Israel Hospital Patient and Family Learning Center will disseminate the information we gain as widely as possible.

Our research agenda includes an evaluation of alternative therapies for: 1) chronic low back pain, 2) childhood ear infections, 3) adult hay fever, 4) postmenopausal hot flashes, and 5) coronary artery disease. We will also conduct meta-analyses of placebo response rates across a variety of medical conditions.

The Beth Israel Center has one other bold objective. We will see if it is feasible to create an alternative medicine consultation service. Imagine a hospital outpatient unit where patients can be referred for advice on alternative medical practices by their primary doctor or subspecialist. Imagine a friend or relative with a chronic or life-threatening illness who has exhausted conventional care and needs to know whether acupuncture will help the pain, whether a macrobiotic diet or Chinese herbs should or should not be used during chemotherapy, and so on. Patients have nowhere to ask such questions. We will try to build a service that provides the answers.

One of my favorite Chinese proverbs says "Zhen jin bu pa huo lian": "Real gold does not fear even the hottest fire." If alternative therapies are effective and safe and capable of saving money, we now have the scientific tools to demonstrate this beyond a shadow of a doubt. If these therapies do not predictably offer relief or are unsafe, we will document this. I hope Beth Israel's Center for Alternative Medicine Research will be a model for other centers and research teams to join us in this work.

David Grimes recently wrote, "Doing everything for everyone is neither tenable nor desirable. What is done should be inspired by compassion and guided by science, and not merely reflect what the market will bear." Medical therapies, whether conventional or alternative, should indeed be inspired by compassion and guided by science. My hunch is that the coming years will see an explosion of knowledge blending conventional and alternative therapies, thereby applying both compassion and science to the care of others.

Boston, Massachusetts
April 1995

Index

acupuncture *(continued)*
  psychological factor in, 77–78
  as remedy for common illnesses, 95
  scientific research on, 94–95,
    116–21, 238
  sensations associated with, 65–66,
    119–20
  specific disorders treated by, 113–16
  texts on, 36n, 46, 87, 113, 171n,
    181n, 211
  theoretical basis of, 61–68
  uses of, 60–78, 95
  as viewed by Western physicians,
    120–21, 167–68
  see also meridians, acupuncture;
    needles, acupuncture; points,
    acupuncture
acupuncture charts, 94
*Acupuncture: From Ancient Art to Modern
  Medicine* (Macdonald), 76n
aerobic exercise, 227
alcohol, avoidance of, 130
alcoholism, 194
All-China Institute of Traditional
  Chinese Medicine, 206
allergies, 116
alopecia areata, 102
amenorrhea, 115
*American Transplant: The Rockefeller
  Foundation and Peking Union
  Medical College, An* (Bullock),
  154n
amyotrophic lateral sclerosis (ALS),
  104–7
analgesia, acupuncture, 67–78
  acceptance of, 149–50, 229
  effectiveness of, 88–89, 113, 120–21,
    232
  Qi Gong used in, 145–46, 216
  as substitute for analgesic drugs,
    67–68
anatomy, human:
  landmarks in, 64
  as system of Yin and Yang, 37–40,
    42–43, 234

An Ding Psychiatric Hospital, 190–96
anesthesia:
  acupuncture, 28, 47
  ether, 149–50
  general, 68, 74
  herbal, 75n
  topical, 99
  see also analgesia, acupuncture
angina pectoris, 143
ankle pain, 114, 116
anterior chamber dimension, 202
antibiotics, 12–13, 57, 131
anxiety:
  as disorder, 128, 172, 190
  levels of, 118
  sexual, 194
appendectomies, 28, 163
appendicitis, 28, 114, 163
Artemisia vulgaris, 63n
arthritis, 93, 114, 116, 200–201, 212
asthma, 98–99, 114, 116, 181, 200,
  209, 212
*Away with All Pests: An English Surgeon
  in People's China, 1954–1969*
  (Horn), 29n
Ayurvedic Medicine, 12

back pain, 114, 116, 185, 186
bacteria, 44–45, 56, 213–14
"bad spirits," 170
baldness, hereditary, 101–2
Barefoot Doctor's Manual, 162
barley, 127
behavioral modification, 152, 197,
  227–28, 234
Beijing Capital Hospital, 105, 157
Beijing Foreign Language Institute, 32,
  33, 103
Beijing Friendship Store, 60, 127
Beijing Institute of Traditional Chinese
  Medicine, 22, 33–34, 60, 61, 80,
  90, 109, 113, 119, 157, 174, 191,
  199, 206, 221
Beijing Medical Journal, 158
Beijing Neurosurgical Institute, 68, 69

medicine, traditional Chinese:
  ancient literature of, 35–36, 46, 87,
    211
  concept of disease in, 51, 55–56
  efficacy of, 87–90, 116–21, 237–38
  forefathers of, 35–36
  immediate vs. long-term cures in,
    111, 113, 132–35
  loss of, 93–94
  Qi as fundamental element of, 29
  relationship between man and nature
    in, 40
  scholars of, 35–36, 152
  scientific investigation of, 231–38
  texts for, 35–36, 46, 87, 160, 161,
    211, 228
  theoretical basis of, 36, 37–39, 40,
    52, 55–59, 127
  Western influences on, 34–50,
    167–68
  Western medicine vs., 11–14,
    134–35, 153–56, 209, 212,
    231–38
  see also acupuncture; herbal
    medicines; massage, Chinese;
    medicine
meditation, 198, 200, 208, 222, 227,
    234
Mencius, 211
Ménière's syndrome, 114
menorrhagia, 115
menstrual cramps, 133
mental illness, 169–96
  ancestors as cause of, 170–71
  cases of, 173–86
  in China vs. U.S., 189–90
  disturbance of Qi as cause of, 170,
    171
  drug therapy for, 192, 193, 195
  family problems and, 183–84, 185
  guilt associated with, 171
  hereditary factors in, 170–71, 193
  sexual problems and, 184–88, 194
  somatization of, 170–72, 184, 189,
    195

  as treated by acupuncture, 172,
    173–74, 176, 178, 193
  as treated by Chinese massage, 172,
    173–74, 176, 178
  as treated by herbal medicines, 172,
    173–74, 176, 178, 192, 193
  as treated in psychiatric hospitals,
    190–96
  Western diagnostic criteria for, 169
  Western treatment of, 192, 193–96
  Yin and Yang as applied to, 170,
    196
  see also specific illnesses
meridians, acupuncture:
  collaterals of, 62
  direction of Qi along, 112–13, 211
  extra, 61, 62
  major and minor, 62
  nerve routes vs., 47, 65
  as physical entities, 47, 119–20
  stagnation of Qi in, 96, 109
  "triple burner," 96
metabolic rate, 200, 213
mind-body interactions, 11, 13, 14,
    133, 170, 221–22, 223, 234
Mind Race, The (Targ and Harary), 149n
mind-sets, 12
Ministry of Public Health, 156, 199,
    206, 209, 226, 227
Ministry of Public Health Statistics,
    92n
mobile medical teams, 159
morning sickness, 115
"mother and son" relationship, 40
moxa, 63
moxibustion, 63, 94, 211
mumps, 115
musculoskeletal problems, 92, 115,
    118, 128, 176–78
mutism, 115
myopia, 115, 116, 202–3
mystics, 223

narcotics, 73
National Academy of Sciences, 29